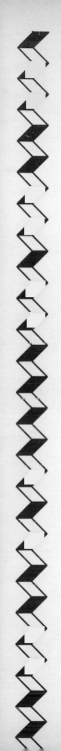

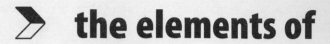 **the elements of**

the chakras

naomi ozaniec

D0288632

ELEMENT

Shaftesbury, Dorset • Boston, Massachusetts • Melbourne, Victoria

© Element Books Limited 1990
Text © Naomi Ozaniec 1990

First published in Great Britain in 1990 by
Element Books Limited

This edition published in 1996
by Element Books Limited
Shaftesbury, Dorset SP7 8BP

Published in the USA in 1991 by
Element Books, Inc.
160 North Washington Street, Boston, MA 02114

Published in Australia in 1991 by
Element Books
and distributed by Penguin Australia Ltd
487 Maroondah Highway, Ringwood, Victoria 3134

Reprinted 1997

Chakra illustrations © Swami Sivananda Radha 1978
Timeless Books, PO Box 50905EB, Palo Alto
CA 94303–0673, USA

Cover design by Max Fairbrother
Typeset by Selectmove Ltd, London
Printed and bound in Great Britain by
Biddles Ltd, Guildford and King's Lynn

British Library Cataloguing in Publication
Data available

Library of Congress Cataloging in Publication
Data available

ISBN 1–86204–029–X

N
ov
w
cl
p

v

OZaniec, naomi?
the chakras,

MEN OF TRINITY
TRINITY EPISCOPAL CHURCH
600 FRANKLIN ST
MICHIGAN CITY, IN 46360

The *Elements of* is a series designed to present high quality introductions to a broad range of essential subjects.

The books are commissioned specifically from experts in their fields. They provide readable and often unique views of the various topics covered, and are therefore of interest both to those who have some knowledge of the subject, as well as to those who are approaching it for the first time.

Many of these concise yet comprehensive books have practical suggestions and exercises which allow personal experience as well as theoretical understanding, and offer a valuable source of information on many important themes.

In the same series

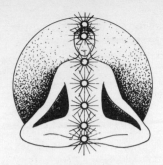

CONTENTS

This book is dedicated to the enlightenment
of all sentient beings.

'The majority of people today live below the diaphragm, and their energies are turned outward into
the material world and prostituted towards material
ends. In the coming centuries this will be corrected;
their energies will be transmuted and purified, and
men will begin to live above the diaphragm. Then
they will express the potencies of the living heart, of
the creative throat, and of the divinely ordered will of
the head.'

The Tibetan[1]

PREFACE

This book came to be written as part of my search for understanding. I needed to make sense of a period in my own life. My chakras were destabilised long before I found a book on the subject, long before I knew that there is a right way and a wrong way to approach the subtle energies. My chakras were worked upon, not by me but by someone else, constituting a prime violation of all the laws of spiritual practice.

I experienced for myself many of the dangers and pitfalls caused by the premature awakening of these energies. This was my baptism by fire, in a literal sense. Time passed, wounds both physical and psychic healed. I found myself left with a burning passion to understand what the chakras have to teach us. I am still asking questions and seeking answers, but I offer the reader what I have gleaned upon the way.

In the spirit of Tantra I have discovered that it is possible to transmute the negative into the positive. It has taken me many years to come to realise this. What has been gained is so much greater than my initial loss. I survived the fiery encounter with the Kundalini serpent. I am glad that I was given such an opportunity in this lifetime. Karma truly equilibrates from one life to another.

Naomi Ozaniec

ACKNOWLEDGEMENTS

I should like to acknowledge all those who helped bring this book to birth. On this plane I would like to thank Jerome who gave me the time to write and Julia McCutchen who read my work so carefully. I would like to thank Timeless Books for their permission to use the line drawings of the chakras and The Theosophical Publishing House who allowed me to quote from the works of Hiroshi Motoyama.

On other planes I must acknowledge and thank the unseen contribution of those guiding minds who always managed to point me in the right direction at critical times.

How to Use This Book

This book is no more than an introduction to a vast area of knowledge. It provides an intellectual framework and some practical guide-lines for working with the energy of the chakras in your own life.

If you decide to implement the exercises indicated, it is absolutely vital that you do not rush through them. Do not anticipate spectacular results. The changes should be gently transformative. You should become more aware of how you draw upon the chakra energies in your life, which ones you spontaneously relate to and which ones seem more distant. Your practice will need to be regular; meditation, pranayama and physical work should ideally become incorporated into your everyday living. This itself is difficult and requires a high level of commitment. What you get from your work will be directly proportional to what you put in.

The book contains sufficient suggestions for you to devise your own programme of work for each of the chakras. You can quite safely combine the affirmations, Bach flower remedies, suitable music and the preliminary exercises. Doing this will orient your mind towards the appropriate chakra. The more advanced techniques of asanas and pranayama are without doubt more demanding. If you feel that these techniques are beyond your capacity or requirement, follow your instincts and wait until you are ready to take on these disciplines.

Ultimate success in this endeavour will depend upon you. The spirit in which you approach this work is critical. Idle curiosity, or pure academic interest will yield only a poor harvest. From the outset you need a deep commitment and the ability to persevere. A book of instruction is in truth a poor substitute for the guidance and insight of a learned teacher as each individual awakens in a unique way, often picking up the threads from previous lives. We do not all start at the same point. Certain people find conscious awakening only too easy; others find it slow, laborious and fraught. Karmic factors are possibly the most significant in determining both our capacity and strength of determination. In the absence of a teacher who might be able to detect the karmic factors involved, it is fair to say that the strength of feeling is a good rough guide of spiritual aspiration. If you have the motivation and willingness to undertake a course of spiritual study and application, you will reap your own reward.

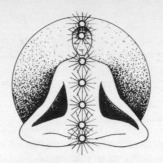

INTRODUCTION

O Goddess! This science of Shiva is a great science. It has always been kept
secret. Therefore, this science revealed by me, the wise should keep secret.

Siva Samhita, verse 206

Our age prizes openness and values unrestricted access to information. Individuals are prepared to fight for the right to know, for the
right to be told and for the right to share information which concerns
their everyday lives. As a society we do not like to feel that any areas
of experience are forbidden, off-limit or restricted. The idea that any
activity should be shrouded in secrecy goes against the democratic
grain. This is truly the age of Everyman and Everywoman.

The subject of this study was kept secret for many centuries.
Knowledge about the chakras was passed from teacher to pupil
as part of an oral spiritual tradition. In this way knowledge was
preserved. Individuals were slowly brought to a full understanding
of the gifts and responsibilities that are inseparable from chakra
awakening. Times change, eventually some aspects of these teachings
were recorded and escaped from the confines of the original lineage.

Our own religious tradition leaves us unprepared to believe that
anything of a spiritual nature could possibly warrant secrecy. Indeed
the exoteric face of religion, with its emphasis on keeping articles of
faith and sharing acts of worship, provides a vehicle which anyone
may join. By contrast the esoteric face of religion offers practice before
doctrine. Esoteric simply means, 'for the few'. It is not a broad path
which invites all. Paradoxically the door to the esoteric path is always
open to all, yet admission is only sought by the few.

Esoteric teachings are commonly thought of as being secret. This
has created an unwarranted air of suspicion and misunderstanding.

1

In reality esoteric knowledge cannot be conveyed in the same manner as other branches of knowledge. If, for instance, I tell you that you have a number of energy centres, or chakras, you may or may not believe me. If you are not convinced by my statement, you will be even less convinced by the arguments that I will muster. If you are inclined to believe me, your acceptance at this stage is no more than intellectual assent. The only way for you really to develop an unshakeable belief in the reality that I have described, is for you to participate actively in your own process of discovery. The discoveries that you make will be entirely personal to you and will depend upon a great number of factors. If you do not wish to test this esoteric hypothesis for yourself, the reality of the chakras will inevitably elude you.

The esoteric path demands your active involvement. You cannot be a bystander or an observer. You must act. When you act in accordance with esoteric principles, and apply esoteric practice, you will create change. No one else can do these things for you. You are in charge of the process.

As the process of total change commences and gathers momentum your attitudes, belief system, values and aspirations naturally undergo radical transformation. This will happen gradually as the process works at its own rate. The process of re-orientation and eventual rebirth is itself secret. It is private, fragile and precious, like the child developing within the protection of the womb. The birth of a new level of consciousness requires the right environment.

The esoteric path interweaves its way through the major religions, surfacing and submerging as external circumstances dictate. The Qabalah presents the inner face of Judaism. The Sufi tradition presents the inner face of Islam. Shignon Buddhism presents the inner way within Japanese Buddhism. Tantra combines the inner paths of both Hinduism and Buddhism. All these traditions, curiously, have a deep understanding of the chakras.

Knowledge about the chakras is now percolating its way into the public domain. As the New Age draws closer this is not really surprising. Today there is a genuine thirst in all matters esoteric. Western society has been built upon the rocky foundations of material gain and external power. Exoteric religion has lost its authority. People are turning back to the ancient, gentler ways in the search for a new moral and ethical direction. There is a genuine desire for spiritual uplift and personal involvement which will not be easily assuaged nor will it evaporate. It is too deeply felt.

Disseminating knowledge in any area brings responsibility, for all knowledge gives power when applied. Esoteric knowledge is no exception. It has the power to change people's lives dramatically. There is safety within the context of a spiritual tradition, which we lose in part when we extract and isolate particular teachings. There are some current teachers who would consider it most unwise to teach anything about the chakras outside the framework of a tradition. A little learning can be a dangerous thing, and a little esoteric learning can be disastrous.

There are certainly some dangers in broadcasting esoteric seeds to the wind. It is impossible to know whether instructions will be observed or whether the reader will simply decide to try a short cut. It is impossible to judge the readiness and suitability of candidates. Both Yoga and Tantra recognise the many different temperaments and types of person who seek teaching. Both systems can draw upon a wide range of approaches in order to match the student to the work. The medium of the written word makes it impossible to give extra help or to foresee all the problems that might ensue. The reader is left alone to analyse and process any changes that result from partaking in the work. Nevertheless this method for disseminating esoteric principles seems to be appropriate for the time and place in which we live. So we will endeavour to make a virtue of it.

We have to balance the potential harm that might result from disseminating this specific aspect of esoteric knowledge against the potential good that might come from it. We also have to give responsibility and credit to the good sense and spiritual maturity of the reader. Anyone involved in their own spiritual awakening through yoga, psychic development or metaphysical training of any kind is already working with the chakras. Anyone working as a medium, a psychic, a healer, or spiritual practitioner of whatever persuasion is also working with these living energies. Knowledge in this instance can be helpful and indeed absolutely necessary at times. There seems to be a general lack of understanding about the chakras even in western esoteric circles. I have often encountered the attitude that chakras are 'eastern things', as if Westerners did not have chakras. Everyone has chakras.

The undeniable spiritual impetus within the west is giving rise to a new tradition which is eclectic and dynamic. This new tradition draws from many sources and incorporates spiritual, psychological and therapeutic aspects. It is keenly focused on the problems of the real world and has a deep commitment to rediscovering spiritual realities. Knowledge of the chakras will surely be safe in these hands; I hope this proves to be so.

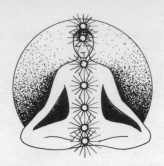

1 · THE LANDSCAPE OF SUBTLE ENERGIES

In your body is the mountain Meru,
Surrounded by the seven continents.
There are streams too,
Lakes, mountains, plains,
And the gods of the various regions.
There are prophets there,
Monks and places of pilgrimage.
And above the ruling gods
There are stars, planets,
And the sun together with the moon;
And there are also the two cosmic powers,
The one that destroys and the one that creates;
And all the elements; ether,
Air and fire, water and earth.
Yes, all these things are within your body;
They exist in three worlds,
And all fulfil their ordered tasks
Around the mountain of Meru.
Only the one who knows this
Can become a true yogi.

Siva Samhita, verses 1–5

'Chakra' is a Sanskrit word meaning wheel. A wheel spins on its own axis; it can turn slowly or rapidly. Like the coloured disks which children spin on a length of thread, a chakra spins in relation to the degree of energy in the system. The wheel itself is a powerful symbol representing the many cyclic patterns of life. It is rather curious to find that this ancient and foreign term is now fully integrated into New Age vocabulary. As so often is the case these days, what appears to be 'New Age', is in reality, extremely 'Old Age'.

Chakras are also called lotuses or padmas. This beautiful symbol tells us a great deal about the nature of the chakra as a living force. The lotus, which is not unlike a water lily, grows widely throughout Asia. The exquisite flower blooms upon the water, but its roots are deeply buried in the mud far below the surface. It has come to represent the human condition. It is rooted in the mud and darkness of the depths but ultimately it flowers under the light of the sun. Just like a lotus, the chakra can be closed, in bud, opening, or blossoming, active or dormant.

The chakras evolve naturally over a long period of time as part of the development of the whole person. Some spiritual systems seek to educate the whole being, knowing that the chakras will change accordingly. It is also possible to quicken the pace of opening and to accelerate this evolutionary process. Other spiritual systems seek to awaken the chakras, knowing that this will accordingly affect the whole being.

Where are the chakras, wheels or lotuses? They are to be found within each of us. Just as everyone has a physical body, so, too does everyone also have a subtle body. The chakras serve as a bridging mechanism between physical matter and subtle matter.

We find information about the chakras most notably in Hindu canonical literature, starting with the Upanishads. Four texts in particular deal with the chakras; the Shri Jabala Darshana Upanishad, the Cudamini Upanishad, the Yoga-Shikka Upanishad and the Shandilya Upanishad. These texts describe the location of the chakras and provide symbolic descriptions for each of them.

In the tenth century the *Gorakshashatakam* was written by the Guru Goraknath. He was widely thought of as a saint in his own time. He set out practical knowledge for the benefit of disciples. His text gave new information concerning the powers that accompany the awakening of the centres. He also established the connection between chakra awakening and the practice of meditation.

We find the most detailed and comprehensive study of the chakras in the *Sat-Cakra-Nirupana* (Description of and Investigation into the Six Bodily Centres). This is the sixth chapter of a major work composed in the sixteenth century by Purananda Svami called

Shri-Tattva-Cintamini and it includes detailed descriptions of the chakras, with illustrations. The text also identifies the powers that accompany the awakening of the chakras and describes the practices which the disciple needs to master. In modern parlance this text has all the qualities of a workbook.

The Hindu tradition is a rich source of information and inspiration. It furnishes us with descriptions, representations and practical techniques for chakra work. The spiritual initiates of this tradition worked extensively with these energies and left a rich heritage of paintings, symbolic images, cosmograms, meditations and texts.

We find teachings concerning the chakras in many other major spiritual traditions. Within Tibetan Buddhism, knowledge of the chakras is thoroughly integrated into practice. The centres are called channel wheels. They are used extensively in certain significant visualisations by the practitioner. Taoist yoga is a complex discipline based upon the control and circulation of vital energies. The western alchemical tradition had a deep understanding of the chakras. Metals and planets were assigned to the chakras in an elaborate system of correspondences that formed the basis of the alchemists' approach to the quest for spiritual transformation. With the decline of the alchemical arts, codified knowledge about the chakras faded in the west.

Interest in the chakras re-emerged with the appearance of the Theosophy movement in the late nineteenth and early twentieth century. Theosophists were especially interested in a wide range of eastern metaphysical concepts and brought many key ideas to western minds. The Theosophical Publishing House produced several volumes on the chakras, the most notable of these being *The Chakras* by C. W. Leadbeater. More recently still we have the collected works of Alice Bailey to draw upon. She was in telepathic communication with the Tibetan master, Djwhal Khul, for some thirty years. The Tibetan gave few personal details during this long period. He vouchedsafed only what is given in the preface to each volume; namely that he lived on the borders of Tibet and defined his task in the following way, 'My work is to teach and spread the knowledge of the Ageless Wisdom wherever I can find a response'. Their fruitful collaboration produced a vast storehouse of esoteric teaching, including a wealth of information on the chakras. We find broad agreement throughout these widely-differing sources concerning the location, nature and function of the chakras.

It is my own personal belief that as the New Age draws closer, changes in group consciousness will bring about a re-evaluation of the chakras and their significance for us individually and as a group. We are entering an age when spiritual values will take on a deep significance at a far wider level. The chakras represent the spiritual blueprint that many will turn to in the quest to find themselves.

THE CHAKRAS AND SUBTLE ANATOMY

The chakras themselves are part of a greater network of subtle energies. We cannot isolate them without violating holistic principles. Our physical make-up is well researched and documented through the many body-based sciences. Our subtle make-up can only be explored through quite different means: involvement rather than clinical detachment, and an holistic frame of reference. However, the physical and the non-physical aspects of being are two aspects of the same whole; they cannot really be separated. We cannot study one without reference to the other. We cannot study subtle anatomy without seeing its relationship to physical anatomy. Equally, physical anatomy without knowledge of subtle anatomy is incomplete.

The idea that living cells, whether in human, animal or vegetable form, radiate an invisible presence has been an enduring concept. The development of Kirlian photography has now revealed the reality of life energy for the first time. It is possible to see energy flows and emanations from quite simple life forms captured in beautiful photographic form. This technique has revealed the reality of non-physical energies quite clearly. If we are now able to catch a glimpse of the emanations from simple cell structures such as plants and even vegetables, we can only wonder what intricate energy patterns conscious and complicated human beings might radiate.[2]

Simple aggregations of living tissue generate a luminescence. It is therefore likely that more specialised groups of cells arranged into physical organs will give rise to more organised energy patterns. Stop for a moment and list the body's major systems. Your list will probably include cognition, respiration, circulation, digestion, reproduction and excretion. Their equivalents are the six chakras of awakening. The brain, not surprisingly, has an additional centre giving a total of seven major chakras. These are located over the top of the head, over the brow at the centre of the forehead, at the throat, at the heart, at the solar plexus, at the sexual centre and at the base of the body (see Fig.1).

THE CHAKRAS AND THE PHYSICAL BODY

Each chakra corresponds to certain physical systems and the related

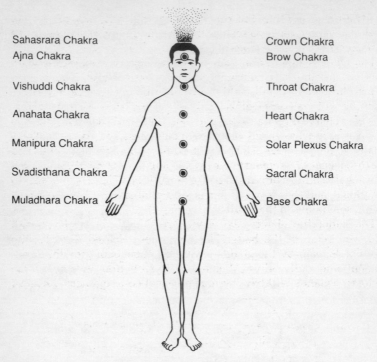

Sahasrara Chakra	Crown Chakra
Ajna Chakra	Brow Chakra
Vishuddi Chakra	Throat Chakra
Anahata Chakra	Heart Chakra
Manipura Chakra	Solar Plexus Chakra
Svadisthana Chakra	Sacral Chakra
Muladhara Chakra	Base Chakra

Figure 1. The Seven Chakras

organs. The base chakra relates to the large intestine and the rectum. It also shares some responsibility for the functions of the kidneys which rid the body of waste matter. The sacral chakra relates to the reproductive system, ovaries and testes, the bladder and the kidneys. The solar plexus chakra relates to the liver, gall bladder, stomach, spleen and small intestine. The heart chakra relates to the heart and the arms. The throat chakra relates to the lungs and throat. The brow chakra relates to the brain. The crown chakra is not limited to one part of the body, but relates to the whole being.

There is a direct relationship between the condition of the chakra and the corresponding physical organs. A chakra can be over-vitalised, under-vitalised or in a state of balance. It can be open or blocked. Dysfunction, for example, of the reproductive system will usually manifest with obvious physical symptoms such as disrupted menstruation. The physical symptoms will be mirrored by dysfunction within the related energy network and the chakra itself. Creating change to restore the related energy system to a state of balance will create change at the physical level.

The chakras function as transmuters of energy from one level to another, distributing pranic energy to the physical body. This is done in part through the glands, which regulate different systems within the body. Traditionally each of the chakras is also related to a major gland. The base chakra is related to the adrenals; the sacral chakra is related to the ovaries in women and the testes in men; the solar plexus chakra is related to the pancreas. The heart chakra is related to the thymus and the throat chakra is related to the thyroid and parathryroid glands. The brow chakra is most often assigned to the pituitary gland, sometimes to the pineal, and the crown chakra is most often assigned to the pineal gland, sometimes to the pituitary (see Fig. 2).

The endocrine glands play a vital role in the everyday health and well-being of the body. The hormones released directly into the bloodstream by the glands govern all aspects of growth, development and daily physical activity. Dysfunction by any of the endocrine glands will have serious physical consequences. Physical

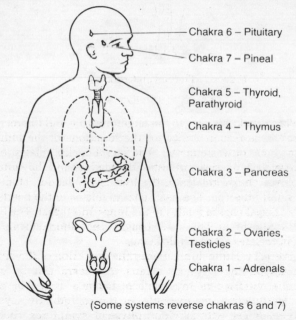

Chakra 6 – Pituitary

Chakra 7 – Pineal

Chakra 5 – Thyroid, Parathyroid

Chakra 4 – Thymus

Chakra 3 – Pancreas

Chakra 2 – Ovaries, Testicles

Chakra 1 – Adrenals

(Some systems reverse chakras 6 and 7)

Figure 2. The Chakras and the Endocrine System

malfunction is itself the result of a breakdown that becomes lodged within the energy network of nadis and chakras.

The number of chakras sometimes varies from one tradition to another. This is not a cause for disagreement but rather a question of accounting. There are two subsidiary centres allied to the heart and throat chakras. Some authorities do not include the centre at the top of the head as a chakra, treating it instead as a unique centre of consciousness. The number of chakras given can therefore vary from six up to nine. The number most often given is seven: the six chakras of awakening and the crown chakra at the top of the head.

The Chakras and the Physical Body

CHAKRA	LOCATION	GLAND
Muladhara	Coccygeal Plexus	Adrenals
Svadisthana	Sacral Plexus	Testes
		Ovaries
Manipura	Solar Plexus	Pancreas
Anahata	Cardiac Plexus	Thymus
Vishuddi	Cervical Plexus	Thyroid
		Parathyroid
Ajna	Cavernous Plexus	Pituitary
Sahasrara	Meridian Plexus	Pineal

THE SUSHUMNA, IDA AND PINGALA MERIDIANS

Just as the physical body is far more than just a collection of organs, the subtle vehicle is far more than a collection of chakras. The physical organs are connected as part of a greater whole, and the chakras are also connected as part of a greater whole. The body has other vital systems without which it could not function: it has a complicated network of nerves, centralised in the spinal column, highly developed senses and a vitally important system of hormone regulators. The subtle vehicle also has other vital systems: there is a network of interconnecting energy channels called meridians or nadis (the word 'nad' means to flow). There are a number of major channels also called meridians and a vast number of increasingly finer minor ones. The *Siva Samhita* states in verse 13 that 'In the body of Man there are 350,000 nadis; of them, the principal are fourteen'.

Within the physical body the spine is of great importance, and the spine also has a vital part to play in the circulation of subtle energies. The sushumna, which is the most important of the nadis, rises within the base chakra following the spine. The Siva Samhita tells us in verse 16 that 'Sushumna alone is the highest and beloved of the Yogis. Other vessels are subordinate to it in the body'. It terminates at the crown chakra, the Gate of Brahman. The sushumna nadi is also known as the channel of fire or Sarasvati, one of India's sacred rivers. Sushumna itself is threefold in nature, containing finer forces arranged one within the other. The innermost of these is citrini, 'The Heavenly Way, this is the giver of the joy of immortality'. This current is equilibrating by nature.

Next comes vajra; its nature is active and forceful. The outer channel is sushmuna; its natural tendency is towards inertia and inactivity. The chakras are rooted upon citrini but open upon the surface of the appropriate energy field. Alice Bailey describes the sushumna as being composed of the forces of life, consciousness and creativity. It bears a remarkable resemblance to the governor vessel meridian which rises at the tip of the coccyx, travels up the centre of the back and passes over the back of the head to finish at the upper lip. This is a major meridian in acupuncture.

In addition to the sushumna there are two other important channels; ida and pingala. Ida is also called chandra, the moon or the Ganges River, while pingala is also known as surya, the sun or the Yamuna river. The pingala nadi emerges from the right side of the base chakra and travels up the body in a series of curves crossing back and forth over the sushumna. The ida nadi emerges from the left side of the base chakra and travels up the body, creating the other half of a symmetrical pattern. Ida, pingala and sushumna meet at the brow centre between the eyebrows and form a plaited knot of energies. From here the three rivers Ganges, Yamuna and Sarasvati flow as a single current. The pattern they make has been likened to a pair of intertwined serpents. Some authorities indicate that ida and pingala form a pattern that passes around the chakras (see Fig. 3). Other authorities, including Swami Saytananda, indicate that the chakras emerge at the junctions where ida and pingala cross sushumna (see Fig.4).

The spiral pattern created by ida and pingala is not mirrored in any of the traditional meridians used in acupuncture. However, Hiroshi Motoyama, a modern researcher and practitioner of the spiritual science, sees a strong correspondence between the second line of the bladder meridian of acupuncture and the ida and pingala nadis. The bladder meridian originates near the bridge of the nose, flows over the head and then courses down the back, dividing into two branches. The second line flows down the back about 4.5cm on either side of

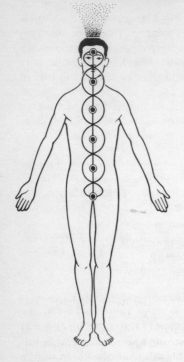 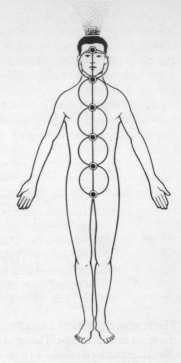

Figure 3. The Route of Ida   Figure 4. An Alternative Route
      and Pingala   for Ida and Pingala

the spine. This meridian is especially important, having points which regulate all the internal organs. However, ida and pingala do not pass over the top of the head and are always represented upon the front of the body. They commence at the base chakra and terminate at the brow. I have puzzled hard over these lines of energy which are not represented by meridians, yet which seem valid as representations of the living energy system.

In my dowsing work I have noted that the left and the right side of a healthy body produce clockwise and counter-clockwise flows of energy. This effect seems to be connected to the polarity of the body, which is primarily established through the two hemispheres of the brain. The chakras fall upon the central line of the body and rotate in various clockwise and counter-clockwise combinations. Moving slightly left of centre (ida) we encounter a swirl moving in a clockwise direction. Moving slightly right of centre we encounter a swirl moving in a counter-clockwise direction. When we combine these two patterns the spiral image naturally emerges as we pass up the body. This same pattern appears as we travel up the back. Any disturbance of this spiral pattern is indicative of the symptoms of localised illness.

Ida and pingala are the polar forces which are generated by the two hemispheres of the brain. This network is anchored at either end of the circuit at the base and brow centres.

THE KUNDALINI EXPERIENCE

> The divine power,
> Kundalini shines
> like the stem of a young lotus;
> like a snake, coiled round upon herself,
> she holds her tail in her mouth
> and lies resting half asleep
> at the base of the body.
>
> Yoga Kundalini Upanishad (1.82)

The spinal network of energies is a vital part of the subtle anatomy of the human individual. The chakras are strung upon the inner column of sushumna like jewels on a necklace. It is this central column which unifies the separated chakras into a whole. It is possible for high levels of energy to rise up from the base chakra through the spinal nadi and dramatically affect all the chakras simultaneously. This force is latent but can be stimulated by work which awakens the chakras individually. The Kundalini force is like a coiled spring. In fact Kundalini is most often depicted in a coiled form as a sleeping serpent. Kundalini shakti can rise and retreat again many times before completing the journey to the top chakra. We cannot understand the chakras individually without considering them as a unified whole, as aspects of a single power.

When the latent power awakens, the ensuing experience takes many forms dependent upon the consciousness of the practitioner. It can be frightening, bewildering, dramatic and disturbing, hardly ever gentle. The full Kundalini experience brings reconstruction of total being. It can be likened to a living second birth with all the accompanying birth trauma. I like to think of it as a quantum leap. I once had a dream in which I saw Kundalini symbolised as a supernova which was described as 'the soul going critical'.

Gopi Krishna's experience of Kundalini was traumatic and devastating. At times he came near to death, at other times he felt that he was losing his sanity. His autobiography, *Kundalini, The Evolutionary Energy in Man*,[3] is compelling and reveals a great deal about the individual chakras. Having taken up Yoga in his quest for truth, he says, 'I longed to attain the condition of consciousness, said to be the ultimate goal of Yoga, which carries the embodied spirit to a region of unspeakable glory and bliss.' After many difficult years he attained his goal, experiencing both glory and bliss. His work is probably the fullest contemporary account of Kundalini's rising. He concluded, 'I am irresistibly led to the conclusion that the human organism is evolving in the direction indicated by mystics, prophets and men of genius, by the action of this wonderful mechanism located at the base of the spine.'

When we are looking at the chakras individually we need to bear in mind the unity represented by the sevenfold nature of the process.

THE AURA

The five senses serve the physical self sufficiently well. Yet esoteric traditions have long taught that both the five senses and the physical form are limited and incomplete expressions of total reality. The physical body is surrounded by an ovoid emanation. It is made up of different bands of energy which each reflect an aspect of being. The innermost band follows the outline of the body. This is the etheric body. Beyond this is a band of finer substance which reflects the emotional nature. It is usually called the astral body or sometimes the desire body. Beyond this still lies the mental body, a level of emanation which reflects the mental nature. Together these bands of energy form the aura, the mirror of being. The aura can be seen through clairvoyant vision in terms of colour, brightness, clarity and definition.

THE ETHERIC FIELD

The belief that we are not purely physical beings is universally held within living spiritual traditions. Such a belief is intimately connected to a wider view of reality. Accordingly the physical form is viewed as one manifestation of total being. It is regarded as the most dense vehicle of consciousness, composed of matter vibrating within certain frequencies. As Kirlian photography has shown us, living cells generate a non-physical luminescence or emanation which interpenetrates and surrounds the organic whole, whether it is vegetable, plant, animal or human. This is the etheric vehicle, sheath, body or field, depending on terminology. It is very easy to feel this energy field through quite basic exercise. This level of vibration is sometimes referred to as the health aura or vital body, as patterns of disease appear first within the etheric form. The physical and etheric levels serve as a unified whole.

The physical sheath is called annamaya kosha in the Upanishads. The etheric vehicle is called pranamaya kosha. Together these two levels are called the atma puri, the city of the soul. Both the physical and the etheric vehicles need prana for the maintenance of health and vitality. The physical body draws mainly upon gross prana provided by food and the air. It also draws upon some degree of subtle prana. The etheric form transmutes subtle prana from more refined levels and transmutes it via the chakras. The etheric level, in contrast to the physical, is highly sensitive to thought patterns, and so the surrounding etheric double can be expanded through visualisation and directed breathing.

THE ASTRAL FIELD

Next we encounter what is commonly called the astral or emotional body. This is also called the desire body as this level reflects our true desires. This band of emanation extends some distance beyond the body in all directions. We might also like to think of it as a system of personal antennae. When we meet someone for the first time, or find ourselves in a strange place, the astral field picks up and transmits sensations to us. We can feel uncomfortable or ill at ease in what appears to be a perfectly acceptable situation. We can sense something about another person long before we are able to confirm this. When two people are attracted, the two energy fields blend or merge by extending towards each other. Conversely, anger and strong feelings of dislike create barriers between the fields: there is no merging or interaction; the two energy fields remain closed.

There is a constant play of energies as the astral field mirrors all changes of mood and responds to the moods and vibrations of others. Human emotions generate specific patterns of energy: hatred, lust, greed, desire, anger, love, devotion – each possesses different vibrations. The astral form reflects the interplay of emotions like a mirror. Its clarity and quality directly reflect the emotional responses. Those with clairvoyant vision indicate that brightness and light accompany the selfless range of emotions such as compassion and altruistic love. The astral sheath can be dark, leaden and even distorted, mirroring persistent ugly emotional states.

The magic mirror is a favourite image in fairy tales. It symbolises the living astral mirror which truthfully reveals desires. The astral field mirrors without discrimination. In children, because the mental field is undeveloped, the astral field opens directly onto the outside world. Adults who have not brought the emotions under mental control remain polarised at this level. If the emotional field is to be aligned to spiritual purpose, a quiet mind, self-awareness and spiritual aspiration need to be nurtured to counter the bias of subjective feeling and the reactive response. Buddhism lays great stress on the development of equanimity as a means of countering the extreme and unbalanced feelings produced by the unrestrained play of the emotions. Personal desires and motives are brought into consciousness and raised to their highest expression through all-embracing compassion. The astral field becomes the mirror for the highest emotions when the emotions that feed the self have been stilled.

THE MENTAL FIELD

The mental sheath constitutes the outer and least dense aspect of the aura. It appears to commence at the edge of the astral field, although in fact it interpenetrates all astral, etheric and physical substance. This band of energy reflects the mental nature and develops with the ability to use the mind in certain ways. The range of mental activities which our society requires through education and work rarely stimulates development at this level. Alice Bailey outlines the types of activity that sharpen the mental aura. She claims that the individual needs to develop the ability to think clearly 'on all matters affecting the race'. This seems a tall order, but it raises all the fundamental questions that most people seek to avoid, and sets the level for abstract thought. The mind has to be focused through the practice of concentration, comprehended through the practice of meditation and raised to its highest through contemplation. With the development of the higher mental faculties, new abilities quicken. These include the ability to receive inspirational thoughts and intuitive ideas from a pool which invariably appears in an external form. Telepathy and other mental phenomena are also more likely to appear under conscious control.

It is in such ways that the development of the higher mind refines the mental sheath.

THE CAUSAL FIELD

The causal field is grounded in spiritual reality. It interpenetrates the individual mental field and also rests in the universal field. This energy serves as a bridge between levels of unity and duality. Human experience is invariably dualised into 'me' and 'not me'. In the classic mystical experience there is an overwhelming sense of oneness. The distinction between 'me' and 'not me' simply does not exist.

The world of matter, intertwined with etheric energies, is a plane of effects. What we see about us does not originate upon this level but results from certain laws. The Qabalah portrays the process of manifestation as a series of emanations. This is very similar to the idea of a hierarchy of increasingly refined and subtle states. The causal level, as its name implies, is a plane of origination, not of manifestation.

The individual human being has little awareness of this level. As we live upon the material plane it would be very difficult for us to maintain this degree of consciousness. Those mystics who have briefly touched this level are often ill-at-ease within the illusions of matter. Nevertheless it is sufficient for us to know that we are rooted into the universal life through the causal field. The causal body is called the anandamaya kosa, or body of bliss.

The subtle energies are just as complicated as the physical form. The key to working with these energies is simple in essence but difficult in application. The subtle energies respond most readily to applied thought. As in the esoteric saying, 'Energy follows thought,' our subtle energies reflect our mental states for good or ill. The axiom also means that habitual attitudes produce equally engrained patterns of energy, which in turn affect our health and well-being. If we wish to create change we have to take charge of ourselves by changing our patterns of consciousness.

The relationship between the physical and subtle energies is complex. The subtle levels of our being indicate hidden levels of potential within us all. If we each possess seven major centres of awakening, it is certain that the vast majority of us have not yet explored the potential that these represent. Our condition can be likened to a person who sits motionless, having yet to discover the functions of physical limbs.

Becoming conscious of our own true nature is a difficult and often painful process. It requires a commitment, freely given, to follow the path towards our own enlightenment. It necessitates working with consciousness and with our own depths. The process requires that we slough off old levels of identification as many times as is necessary. This is the ageless Quest for Ultimate Reality. It takes many forms and is at the heart of all true spiritual practice. The Tibetan reminds us of the difficulty of the path: 'No glamour, no illusion can long hold the man who has set himself the task of treading the razor-edged Path which leads through the wilderness, through the thick-set forest, through the deep waters of sorrow and distress, through the valley of sacrifice and over the mountains of vision, to the gate of Deliverance.'[4] Fortunately, should we set out on the quest, we will not travel empty-handed. The way has been mapped out by previous quest-seekers, who have bequeathed their treasure; the Yoga of the east or the Yoga of the west, the Qabalah.

The Qabalah means 'from mouth to ear', indicating that it was originally an oral tradition. Like all esoteric traditions, its followers were subject to persecution. The Judaic tradition, however, created an image, a symbolic picture to serve as the focal point for the transmission of its teachings. This is the Otz Chim, the Tree of Life, shown in Fig. 5.

This unique symbol functions at many levels simultaneously. It is depicted as a series of ten spheres, with an additional veiled eleventh sphere and twenty-two interconnecting paths which are like branches. Together the spheres, which are called sephiroth, and the paths describe the universal forces of the macrocosm and the microcosm.

Maps of the quest, like any decent guide book to a new country, provide the traveller with a route, a method, instructions for protection, knowledge of certain landmarks along the way and possible dangers that might be encountered. The vital difference is that you are both the traveller and the path, the journey and the goal. The value of such maps is beyond measure. Spiritual knowledge is sometimes described as treasure. This theme typically occurs in fairy tales where the hero sets out on the quest and faces many dangers before he wins the treasure, which is often buried and is usually guarded by a fearsome beast. In defeating the guardian, the hero or candidate successfully earns the right to obtain the treasure.

The quest of the hero is often parallelled in real life by a conscious search for the keys to inner discovery. This takes many forms: study, reflective thought, deep conversation, personal commitment, or active

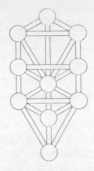

Figure 5. The Tree of Life – Otz Chim.

participation in a spiritually orientated group of like minds. At few other times in history has the way to this treasure been so open and accessible at a mass level. Previous questers had to undertake the search in a literal sense. The Tantric document already mentioned, *Sat-Cakra-Nirupana*, translated by Sir John Woodroffe, was a closely-guarded secret even in India. For a long time it was believed that the work had perished. It took Sir John Woodroffe half a lifetime of patient searching to locate it and further years of dedicated work to translate it. Another text, *The Secret of the Golden Flower*, was transmitted orally within a small esoteric tradition in China for many centuries. It was not committed to paper at all until the eighteenth century. Then in 1920 one thousand copies were made and distributed to a small group. Richard Wilhelm came across a copy and recognised its value. He undertook the painstaking task of translating it for a western audience.

We are left to wonder what other significant texts have been lost, deliberately destroyed or forgotten. Every person who takes up the challenge of the quest becomes in essence a new book and ensures that this special knowledge is in safe keeping for the next generation.

DISCOVERING THE ETHERIC FIELD

Position your hands so that they are facing but not touching each other. You may need to experiment with the distance as there is definitely a critical point at which the energy centres in the palms interact with one another. Begin to move your hands slowly in and out from each other in a bouncing movement. You might already begin to feel something at this point. When the two palm centres interact you will feel what can best be described as a magnetic force between your hands. This is quite different from the experience of general body heat. When you discover this sensation, which cannot be mistaken, you can begin to move the hands slightly further apart. Eventually the contact will be broken as you move beyond the reach of your own energy field.

You can intensify the experience by breathing slowly and rhythmically. On the outbreath visualise white light pouring out from the palms. When you have mastered this exercise you can go on to refine your sensitivity by bouncing the fingertips of one hand off the palm of the other hand. Do this with your eyes closed to develop your other senses. You can also try this with another person. Energy can be sent by one person and received by the other. If you are sending energy your hands will become quite cold; if you are receiving energy you will feel warmth in the localised area. A great deal can be learned from these very simple exercises.

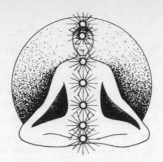

2 · APPROACHING THE GATES

Discover the serpent of illusion by the help of the serpent of wisdom and then will the sleeping serpent mount upwards to the place of meeting.

The Tibetan[1]

The recent interest in chakra awakening presents us with something of a problem. The west does not have a recognised system for the transmission of this specialised knowledge. In the east knowledge about the chakras is integrated in the tantric teachings of Tibetan Buddhism and in the Kundalini Yoga of Hinduism. It is firmly based within sacred tradition and within the close bond of the teacher-pupil relationship.

We in the west must attempt to turn our disadvantage into opportunity. We do not have the strength found in linear transmission or the security of spiritual teachers close at hand. We do however enjoy a freedom of approach and we are not restricted by age-old tradition. We are free to explore and discover for ourselves because we do not have a rule book to follow. We may of course simply rediscover what the east has long known and documented, but at least we can experience the discovery for ourselves. As we approach the chakras we would do well to take the traditional views and methodology into account, for it would be foolish to ignore the accumulated wisdom of the centuries. We do not want to be the fools who rush in where angels fear to tread.

In *A Treatise on White Magic* by Alice Bailey, the Tibetan provides us with a working guideline for awakening the chakras. The first essential requirement on the part of a student is character building. This places chakra awakening firmly in the context of daily life and places responsibility directly upon the individual. The Tibetan asks that we examine ourselves to discover the forces that dominate our lives so that we may consciously seek to redress any obvious imbalance. We are asked to 're-organise, re-orientate and rebuild' the very essence of our being.[2] This is no different from the requirement demanded of the candidate at the portal of the mysteries. The age-old injunction, 'Know thyself' is still the key to admission into the spiritual life. The traditional discipline of Yoga also demands a long period of preparation and ethical reorientation.

The would-be student is therefore asked by the Tibetan to follow the five aspects of Yama, or abstention from evil conduct. These are non violence, truthfulness, sexual continence during certain periods, non-stealing and non-greed. The student is also asked to follow the five aspects of Niyama, or virtuous conduct. These are purification, contentment, asceticism, the recitation of sacred sounds, and the worship of divine beings. Yama and Niyama together prepare the mind for enlightenment. This period of re-orientation is considered to be absolutely essential. It is like preparing the ground in readiness for the seed. The western student could likewise benefit from such a period of preparation.

The Tibetan next asks that we examine our motives for seeking chakra awakening. There has to be a genuine commitment to self-discovery and realisation. Anything less will be insufficient to sustain the individual through the inevitable trials and difficulties of the path. The right motive is essential at the outset. The wrong motive will bring only disappointment.

After examining our motives for seeking to awaken the chakras, we are asked to examine our commitment to the principle of service. It is important that we should genuinely wish to give the benefits of our awakening for others in some way. Right motivation will naturally lead to a commitment to service. Wrong motivation will create the desire to wield power rather than to offer service. The principle of service is also deeply enshrined within those western mysteries that uphold the motto, 'To know in order to serve.'

These first three requirements mark a period of preparation and underline the significance of the decision to awaken the centres. By seeking to work with the energies of the chakras we are seeking to discover ourselves. The next three requirements cover the practical application of this commitment. The practice of meditation is recommended to those students who are securely grounded in the stability of the initial requirements. Meditation is a primary tool in all areas of spiritual awakening. It was Goraknath who first commended meditation as a means of activating the chakras in his treatise written in the tenth century. The practitioner uses the many symbols and qualities of the chakras as focal points for meditative practice. Meditation is an essential approach for chakra awakening, which cannot safely take place without the states of mind implicit in meditation.

The student is next asked to gain a working knowledge of the centres through intellectual study. This entails gaining an overall understanding of the names, location, function and inter-relation-ships between the chakras. According to the Tibetan this will lead naturally to an appreciation of the vibration, colour, tone and astrological significance of the centres. After the student has created an intellectual framework for personal work, the study of the applied breath, pranayama is recommended as the second practical technique.

The Tibetan's guidelines are eminently applicable for any modern student seeking to work with the energies of the chakras. Yoga, for example, offers a thoroughly integrated system for awakening the chakras. With Yoga, the initial period of preparation is followed by gradual absorption of the techniques of pranayama, meditation and physical asanas or postures. The postures function at many levels. They have an obvious effect upon physical well-being by releasing muscle tension, strengthening internal systems and releasing stiffness in the joints. The asanas also have an impact upon the etheric levels by working upon the nadis, which circulate the subtle energies. When combined with certain states of mind, Yoga also affects the astral and mental levels of being by bringing calmness and control.

Hiroshi Motoyama has allocated a series of postures specifically to the chakras (see Appendix 1). These are organised into two groups. The first group serves as preparatory postures which increase the absorption of prana into the body and regulate the flow. The second group strengthens the sushumna and facilitates the flow of prana through this vital nadi. Those already studying Yoga will be familiar with these postures. Those who wish to work with these postures will find thorough explanations in books such as *Light on Yoga* by B. K. S. Iyengar.

The subtle energies are highly responsive to controlled breathing. Prana can be directed by regulated breathing under the control of specific visualisation. Iyengar tells us that pranayama 'causes the Kundalini to uncoil. The serpent lifts its head, enters the sushumna and is forced up through the chakras one by one to the sahasrara.'[3] Different breathing patterns create different effects upon the subtle energies. Controlled breathing is quite different from the often shallow and unconscious rhythms of our daily life. Pranayama begins with the development of yogic breathing. Pranayama should take place in a well-ventilated room. It should not be practised on a full stomach or bladder, and the body should be relaxed. Retain the breath as long as is comfortable. Over time, the capacity to hold the breath under control will increase. The classic lotus position is ideal for pranayama practice. However, this posture will be beyond the ability of many Westerners. Instead sit so that the spine is straight.

YOGIC BREATHING

The Yogic breath is a synthesis of three breaths. It has three parts as air is taken into the abdomen, the chest and then the nasal passages. This is a very calming breath. It also has the power to release tension and bring a sense of wholeness.

1. Inhale deeply.
2. Let the air fill your abdomen. Feel the expansion within your abdomen as the diaphragm stretches.
3. Let the air fill your chest area. Feel your rib cage expand.
4. Let the air move into your throat and nasal passages.
5. On exhalation empty your nasal passages first, then your chest, finally your abdomen.

In this exercise it is important to move the air smoothly and without a break. There should be no separation between inhalation and exhalation.

THE LOCKS

The word bandha means to hold or to tighten. In the locks various parts of the body are gently but firmly contracted. The locks have an effect upon the flow of prana. There are three locks; the neck or chin lock, the diaphragm lock and base lock. These combine breath control with physical control. The bandhas also help release the granthis or psychic knots which impede the flow of prana through the sushumna.

1. The Neck Lock (Jalandhara Bandha)
This lock releases energy blocked in the region of the upper chest. It

creates space in the upper spine and breaks up bodily tensions which build up as a result of concerted mental activity.

1. Sit with a straight back. Place your palms on your knees.
2. Inhale deeply and hold your breath.
3. Bend your head forwards. Pull in your chin and contract your neck. Pull your shoulders up so that your head is resting on the shoulder muscles. Straighten your arms and lock the elbows.
4. Keep your head centred and lock the posture. Retain the breath comfortably. Exhale and release the lock.

Repeat the lock three times.

2. The Diaphragm Lock (Uddiyana Bandha)

This lock stimulates the solar plexus chakra. As this is the distribution centre for prana throughout the body this lock improves the spread of prana generally.

1. Sit with a straight back. Place your palms on your knees.
2. Exhale deeply, emptying your abdomen and chest.
3. Lift your diaphragm. Pull the organs of the upper abdomen up and back towards your spine.
4. Lock the posture. Hold while it is comfortable. Release and inhale.

3. The Root Lock (Mulabandha)

This is the most complex of the locks. It has a powerful effect on the energies at the base of the spine. It can also release creative energies.

1. Sit with straight back. Place your hands on your knees.
2. Exhale deeply. Contract the muscles of your perineum and draw them upwards.
3. Draw in the lower abdomen towards the spine.
4. Hold the lock while it is comfortable. Release and inhale. Repeat.

The breath is a profound tool for creating physical, emotional and intellectual change. The breathing pattern mirrors the way in which the individual interacts with the world and with himself or herself. It is frequently shallow and incomplete. The traditional breathing patterns, including alternate nostril breathing, hara breathing and the breath of fire can have dynamic effects. These exercises work upon the physical body by increasing the supply of oxygen—which assists the detoxification process—and directly upon the energies of the subtle fields.

ALTERNATE NOSTRIL BREATHING

Stage 1

1. Sit straight with your hands on your knees. Place your right hand on your forehead and place your middle and index fingers between your eyebrows. The thumb is placed by the right nostril and the ring finger is placed by the left nostril.
2. Close your right nostril with the thumb.
3. Inhale, then exhale through the left nostril five times.
4. Release your right nostril and press your left nostril with the ring finger. Inhale, then exhale through the right nostril five times.
   This completes one cycle. Practise until twenty-five cycles can be performed.

Stage 2

1. Close the right nostril with your thumb and inhale through the left.
2. After inhalation, close the left nostril, release the right nostril and exhale out through it.
3. Inhale through the right nostril and close it at the end of the inhalation. Open the left nostril and exhale.

This completes one cycle. The lengths of the inhalation and exhalation should be equal.

Stage 3

1. Close your right nostril and inhale through the left. At the end of the inhalation, close both nostrils and retain the breath.
2. Exhale through your right nostril and then inhale through it keeping your left nostril closed.
3. Close both nostrils and retain the breath.
4. Open your left nostril and exhale through it.

This completes one cycle. Each action: inhalation, retention and exhalation, should be performed to the count of five. Practise until twenty-five cycles can be performed.

Refinements of this exercise later include altering the ratio between times of inhalation, retention and exhalation to produce a final ratio of 1:8:6. This exercise is worth the hard work that is required to master it. Each stage should be practised over a period of months until the procedure has been completely integrated. This practice clears the nadis, brings calmness of mind and increases the supply of oxygen to the blood. It brings awareness of the hot and cold solar and lunar currents carried by the breath.

THE BELLOWS BREATH OR BREATH OF FIRE

1. Sit straight with hands on your knees.
2. Place the right hand on the forehead with the middle fingers between the eyes. Place your thumb beside the right nostril and your ring finger beside the left nostril.
3. Close the right nostril with your thumb. Breathe rapidly and rhythmically through the left nostril twenty times, expanding and contracting the abdomen.
4. Close both nostrils and perform mulabanda or jalandhara.
5. Close the left nostril and breathe twenty times with quick but rhythmical expansions and contractions of the abdomen.
6. Inhale, close both nostrils and perform jalandhara or mulabanda.
This completes one cycle. Perform three cycles.

The bellows breath clears the lungs. It stimulates the appetite and digestion. This is a powerful technique for awakening Kundalini. It should not be practised by people with high blood pressure or heart conditions. It should not be done on a full stomach. This is a vigorous exercise and you may feel a surge of pranic energy shooting up the spine. This may make you feel a little light-headed but there should be no feelings of faintness or excessive giddiness.

PSYCHIC BREATHING

By contrast this is a very quiet and gentle breath. It may be practised for long periods in conjunction with meditation techniques. It produces a calming effect on the nervous system.
1. Close the glottis at the back of your throat.
2. Breathe deeply and softly. This produces a slight snoring sound.

The combination of mind control and breath control should make it increasingly possible to direct prana throughout the body or even outside the body where it can be used to heal another person. Sensitivity to prana will increase with practice. It can be experienced as a sensation of movement or through a sudden change in localised body temperature. The inner eye will also become attuned to the flow of prana which appears to the mind's eye as flecks of brightness, shining filaments of white light, or showers of sparks. Techniques which combine breath control and visualisation help this process considerably.

CIRCULATION OF LIGHT

1. Sit with a straight spine.
2. Imagine a reservoir or pool of light at the base of your spine.
3. Inhale slowly and deeply (use the psychic breath). As you do so draw energy in the form of light up from the base chakra. Let it rise up through the sushumna to the top of your head. When it reaches the top of the head see a cascade of light fountaining out through the head.
4. Let this light circulate on either side of your body and be drawn in again at the base chakra.

This completes one cycle. Perform five cycles.

THE INNER SPIRALS

These exercises develop the awareness of the psychic pathways between the muladhara and the ajna centres.

1. Sit straight with hands on your knees.
2. Become aware of the muladhara chakra at the base of your spine.
3. See the pranic channel starting at the right of the chakra. See it curving out towards the right of the body before it curves back to the left to cross the sushumna at the svadisthana chakra.
4. It emerges on the left side of the body from the mid-line and curves back to cross the sushumna at the solar plexus chakra.
5. It emerges on the right side of the body to curve back to the left before it sweeps back to pass at the heart centre.
6. It emerges on the left and then swings back to cross the sushumna to pass beneath at the throat chakra.
7. It emerges on the right of centre from where it flows into the ajna chakra at the centre point on the sushumna.

The prana will descend via the alternative spiral route.

1. Visualise the ajna chakra between your eyebrows. See the pranic current starting at the right side just above your right nostril.
2. See this channel flowing out over the right cheek. It then turns leftwards before it crosses the sushumna at the mid-line and passes at the throat chakra.
3. It emerges from the mid-line moving towards the left, before it curves back towards the right and crosses the mid-line at the sushumna passing at the heart chakra.
4. It emerges to the right side of the body, then curves back to the mid-line crossing the sushumna at the solar plexus chakra.

5. It emerges towards the left side of the body, and curves back to cross the sushumna at the sacral chakra.
6. It emerges to the right before curving again to cross the sushumna at the base chakra.
7. It emerges upon the left and then curves to the right to enter the base chakra.

This is quite a difficult exercise which can be broken down into at least two parts.

There are many more traditional exercises of this kind which cover the awakening of prana, its expansion, contraction and localisation within particular body parts. It is said that some people are able to see and move prana very rapidly. Others find it a slower process requiring patience and determination. Since such exercises have to be repeated over and over again, right motivation is the greatest sustaining factor when no progress is apparent.

The traditional methods for awakening the subtle energies are breath control, meditation and physical postures. Together these three aspects constitute an integrated approach to working with the centres. No serious student can expect to avoid any of these disciplines.

There are some striking similarities between eastern and western systems. Kundalini Yoga is a specialised branch of Yoga which has concentrated upon subtle energies. It has produced both a theory of subtle anatomy and an integrated methodology for awakening the centres. The Qabalah offers a blueprint which can be unfolded through meditation, ritual and spiritual practice, even though it lacks an integrated physical discipline equivalent to the graded asanas of Yoga. The chakras are activated indirectly as a result of the overall awakening process.

The Qabalah was never intended to be a guide for chakra awakening and we should not expect it specifically to fulfil that function. Nevertheless the attributions assigned to the various sephiroth can be related to the characteristics of the chakras. Kether the Crown automatically equates to the crown chakra. The spiritual experience of Kether is union with God. Binah and Hokmah, Wisdom and Understanding, together equate to the brow chakra. Daath the veiled sephirah, straddling the abyss corresponds to the throat chakra. The heart chakra is represented by Tiphareth, Beauty. Geburah the sphere of Severity and Chesed the sphere of Mercy are also reflected in the workings of the heart chakra. The solar plexus chakra equates to Hod, the sphere of thoughts, and Netzach, the sphere of the emotions. Yesod, rich in lunar and water symbolism, equates to the sacral chakra. Finally Malkuth, the Kingdom, equates to the base chakra (see Fig. 6). This framework provides a structure of comparison across the two systems.

The west offers many theraputic approaches that draw upon knowledge of the chakras. Those working directly in these areas are increasing the pool of available knowledge and helping to construct an integrated body/mind theory.

The chakras are excellent indicators of well-being. When a chakra is blocked or closed the individual is no longer able to access the corresponding energies. The relationship between the physical and supra-physical energies is reciprocal and circular. Imbalance at one level is reflected by imbalance at another. Cause and effect are constantly moving in the ever-changing interplay of physical and etheric energies. We can therefore use the chakras as a means of diagnosis.

It is possible to assess the state of individual chakras by dowsing

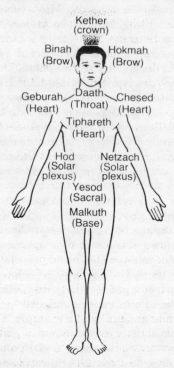

Figure 6. The Chakras and the Tree of Life

with a pendulum. Dowsing can be thought of as a means of amplifying a response which is normally below the threshold of consciousness. We are unconsciously able to relate to many different vibrations generated by varying forms. Organic life, plants, minerals and animate beings all generate energy fields which extend beyond the physical structure. The book that first fired my interest in dowsing is *E.S.P. Beyond Time and Distance* by T. C. Lethbridge. Dowsing is a skill which is best acquired through experience. It is the easiest thing in the world to construct a pendulum from a ring and a length of thread, suspend it over a variety of objects and observe your own deep reaction to the energy system magnified by the pendulum. Experienced dowsers might like to try chakra dowsing for themselves. It is best if the person having a chakra reading lies down flat on their back. The person dowsing can kneel beside them. The pendulum should be suspended over the general area of the chakra, and slowly lowered until it connects with the energy field of the individual. This will vary from person to person. When the pendulum connects with the chakra it will begin to rotate in either a clockwise or an anti-clockwise direction. It will describe a circle, which seems to indicate the circumference of the chakra itself. The speed of rotation is also indicative of the activity of the chakra. The pendulum can be sluggish on occasion or surprisingly rapid. Circular rotation in either direction is indicative of activity and vitality within the chakra. It is more common to find chakras which rotate in a clockwise direction. Physical illness, mirrored within the activity of the relevant chakra, produces either a linear movement of the pendulum or even produces no activity at all, which means the chakra has closed for a while. Dowsing in this way can be illuminating. It shows us very clearly the nature of the relationship between the physical and the etheric levels. A great deal more can be learned about this interface using simple observation skills and dowsing techniques.

The body operates as a hologram, the whole being reflected in the parts. The therapeutic disciplines of acupuncture, reflexology and massage each demonstrates the principle that the body mirrors wholeness within its parts: 'As above so below.' We can therefore locate points in the hands and feet that correspond to the chakras. The reflex points for the pituitary gland assigned to the brow chakra are located on the thumbs and big toes for example. A skilled practitioner can use these points both for diagnosis and as part of treatment.

Working with energy meridians or nodal points requires training and skill if it is to be successful. However, anyone may try the following test; it is taken from the Touch for Health system which is based upon applied kinesiology, the science of muscle activation. Muscle testing provides the basis for all touch for health techniques. The relative strengths of the chakras can also be assessed in this way. It is very easy to do and gives a rough and ready assessment. The test requires two people, the testee and the tester. The testee stands with right arm outstretched with palm down; the left hand is placed over the chakras one at a time. The tester applies a firm downwards pressure to the outstretched arm. The testee is asked to resist as each of the chakras is tested in turn. This test is most interesting. It is impossible to cheat for, try as you might, if a chakra is weak you will not be able to hold out against the pressure from your friend.

There is an even simpler version of this test. The testee connects the tip of the right index finger to the tip of the right thumb. The left hand is placed over the chakras one at a time. The tester tries to pull the testee's thumb and finger apart. It is especially helpful to apply a test to assess the strength of a chakra when you are unwell. There is a great deal to be learned at an individual level by matching patterns of physical illness with patterns of etheric disturbance. You can learn to detect the point of recovery, when the energies flow normally through the related chakra. This point often precedes physical recovery.

The chakras are also highly responsive to approaches, such as the Bach flower remedies, that work specifically upon the subtle energies. The right remedy can have an extraordinarily liberating effect upon a blocked chakra. As the Bach flower remedies are quite harmless it is safe to experiment with them in conjunction with chakra work, and they also work well in conjunction with other intensive approaches.

My attention has been drawn quite recently to a set of gem elixirs. These are potentised mineral preparations. The gem elixirs work directly upon the subtle energies and upon the chakras. My own work with these remedies has so far been limited but favourable.[4]

Deliberate work upon a chakra usually has an impact. Sometimes it is obvious, especially if the individual concerned is sensitive and the results are overt. At other times progress seems slow and the results appear in diffuse forms, new attitudes and new levels of awareness. Chakra work often produces highly symbolic and charged dreams which reveal the condition of the relevant chakra. Dreaming itself can be used as a vehicle for chakra work if the individual is sufficiently attuned to their own dream processes. Dream work can be used as part of an overall strategy for chakra awakening. If you wish to incubate a dream you will need to spend the time before sleeping immersed in the relevant images and thoughts. You will also need to develop the ability to recall your dream images as you wake.

Chakras are highly sensitive to deliberate thought patterns. Affirmations for each chakra are a good way of keeping intentions focused as we go about daily life (see Appendix 2). Create your own affirmations based on these suggestions. Let your affirmation be simple and let it be positive. The affirmation should summarise what the chakra means for you. These positive self-created affirmations can act as a powerful antidote to the endless negative affirmations projected upon us by adults and authority figures as we grow up. How much better to affirm that 'I have the freedom to create my own reality,' than constantly to be told, 'You can't do that.' The affirmation can be used like a meditation while you are working with one chakra. It can be repeated aloud or used silently. It is also a good idea to write down the affirmation and take it with you wherever you go. This simple act merely serves to remind you of its value. The affirmation is best used in conjunction with a dynamic approach.

One of the simplest and most illuminating ways of connecting with the chakras is simply to allow the inner mind to provide symbols and images for each of the chakras. Prepare by assembling a wide range of colours in any medium that you wish. Take a large sheet of paper and enter a quiet meditative state. Attune yourself to each of the chakras in turn and simply draw the images that come to mind. This exercise is quite fascinating. Dark, sombre colours inevitably reveal the inability to express the energy of a particular chakra. Organic shapes and flowing lines indicate harmony and ease of expression. Integration or separation reveals itself in the form and degree of connections between the chakras. The relative size of individual chakras and their emphasis in the whole pattern reveals the degree of spontaneous use.

Having some measure of the overall interaction of the chakras at any given moment is important as we begin to operate more consciously with the energies. We might like to work on a chakra that feels blocked and inaccessible. We might like to work with a physical symptom by engaging the energy that underpins it. We might simply like to have some way of observing the effects of our conscious interaction with chakra energy. Experiment with the approaches suggested, develop a way that comes naturally to you and make it part of your life. There is one golden rule, however, when it comes to work of this nature. If you experience dramatic results that make you feel unstable or off-balance, stop! Do not apply any further pressure. Try to rest and allow the energies to stabilise. This is especially important if you are working on your own. In mystery tradition it is said, 'Make haste slowly.'

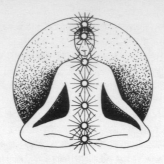

3 · THE KEYS TO THE CHAKRAS

That Gnosis from which the speech and mind turn back baffled, is only obtained through practice; for then this pure Gnosis bursts forth of itself.

The Siva Samhita, verse 180

If a picture is worth a thousand words then a symbolic picture is worth words beyond number. A symbol is open ended; it expands the mind and allows ideas to roam, to free associate, and to gel into newly-formed patterns. Universal symbols retain power across the centuries. Undiminished by the passing of time and undimmed by changing values, these symbols have the capacity to awaken each new generation.

Words are often restrictive. I can pass information to you through words. I can tell you about the chakras. Yet words alone will not initiate you into the inner meaning of the chakras. You are the only person able to do this by inwardly absorbing the attributes, qualities and functions of the chakras through meditation and active participation.

Each chakra is symbolically described by a system of correspondences. The chakras are allocated to colours, geometric shapes (yantras), sounds (mantras), elements, animal symbols and presiding deities. Each chakra is also described as having a particular number of petals. These have been said to represent the vibration of each chakra. Others have suggested that these numbers refer to the spinal nerves related to each plexus. The Tibetan tells us that the word 'petal' only symbolises an expression of force. Sanskrit letters are also allocated to each of the chakras.

These symbolic descriptions can be thought of as a shorthand or code that summarises the essential qualities of the chakra. A symbol can be thought of as a door. It remains tightly shut unless you have the right key.

The chakra images convey little if you just look at them. You need to internalise the forms through meditation. Then the door will swing open easily. You will understand not merely the appearance but the meaning of each of the symbolic representations.

The representations of the chakras that were developed within the Hindu framework are effective, informative and powerful. However, these images are not the only possible means of symbolising these energies. We have plenty of alternative symbolic pictures from within the Indian tradition itself. One version that depicts the manipura chakra shows the presiding deity with his Sakti being carried upon a mythical bird. An eighteenth century gouache on paper from Rajastan depicts the chakras as abstract vortices of ascending energy. Other traditions employ different images. This should give us the courage to create our own images for the powers of the chakras.

Let us now look at the traditional symbols. Each of the chakras is now commonly assigned to a specific colour. This system of colour attribution does not exist in the *Sat-Cakra-Nirupana*. It would seem to be a late addition, probably of western origin. Accordingly, the chakras are assigned to the colours of the rainbow: red, orange, yellow, green, blue, indigo and violet. This does not mean that the chakras themselves are these colours. The colours indicate the relative vibration of the chakras, moving from the slowest at the base to the most rapid at the top of the head. The colours themselves also carry certain symbolic values which the western mind easily comprehends. Red is strong and forceful; orange is less aggressive but nevertheless fiery; yellow is solar and warming; green is cool and promotes natural growth; blue is the colour of healing; indigo is expansive; violet is associated with spiritual aspiration.

The traditional chakra images are also coloured according to a specific code indicated in the *Sat-Cakra-Nirupana*. The colour of the petals, the letters inscribed on them and the yantra attributed to each chakra, are all assigned to specific colours. These also carry symbolic values. The yellow square of privithi, the yantra of the base chakra, signifies elemental earth. The crescent moon, yantra of the sacral chakra, is white signifying elemental water. The triangle, yantra of the solar plexus chakra, is red signifying elemental fire. The hexagon of the heart chakra is a smoky green, signifying the element of air. The circular yantra of the vishuddi chakra is again white. The ajna chakra is predominantly white. It does not have a yantra. This colour is associated with the coolness of the moon and Nirvana. The Sahasrara is not described either in terms of colour or a yantra.

It is only too easy to become swamped by these details and to lose sight of the essentials. Colour symbolism can only be informative when related to its own cultural background. Eastern and western systems attribute quite different meanings to the same colours. Both systems can be used independently of each other. It is a mistake to think that one system is right and the other is therefore wrong. Both systems work in themselves. It is important to remember that these colours do not describe the actual chakras but represent the attempt to convey the qualities associated with the chakras.

The Chakras: Colours

CHAKRA	PETALS	LETTERS	YANTRA
Base	Crimson	Gold	Yellow
Sacral	Vermilion	Lightning	White
Solar Plexus	Blue-green	Blue	Red
Heart	Vermilion	Vermilion	Smoky
Throat	Smoky purple	Red	White
Brow	White	White	White

Each of the chakras is also assigned to an element. This links the qualities of the chakra to a constellation of ideas which are represented by the elemental qualities. The element of earth, attributed to the base chakra, does not refer solely to physical earth. It refers to the qualities of being which might also be thought of as earthy in themselves: practicality, survival, organisation and structure. Earth is slow to change, it has to be manipulated. It is fertile but requires labour; it is our provider and mother.

In the same way the element of water, attributed to the sacral chakra, refers to qualities which could be said to be of a watery nature: reflection, movement, flow and depth. Water has no shape of its own; it is passive in relation to its surroundings. It cleanses and revives. Our bodies contain and require water; life begins in the womb. The menstrual cycle is closely connected to the lunar cycle. There is a close connection between all waters and the influence of the moon.

The element of fire is assigned to the solar plexus chakra. It includes those qualities that might be thought fiery: action, change, expansion and passion. Fire is difficult to confine. It is expansive and volatile. It warms and comforts. Metabolic change generates warmth. When our stomachs are empty we are cold. Fire has the power to change things from one state to another. Fire is always active but it needs constantly to be fuelled.

Elemental air, attributed to the heart chakra, refers to those qualities that might be termed airy by nature: pervasion, omnipresence and invisibility. Air cannot be seen; we cannot touch air yet it touches us; it can be seen only through its effect. Winds circulate around our planet in huge patterns affecting us all. Air is never still; it is active. It is unlimited and shared by everyone.

Akasa is also called ether or spirit. This element is attributed to the throat chakra. It refers to the eternal undying qualities that underlie all manifest forms. Its outer form might be thought of as prana, the universal life force. Akasa is beyond both space and time. It represents a mystery.

Neither the brow nor crown chakras are attributed to any particular elements by tradition. Anodea Judith, writing in *Wheels of Life*, attributes light to the brow chakra and thought to the crown chakra. The elemental attributions are best comprehended through meditation.

The Chakras: the Elements

CHAKRA	ELEMENT
Base	Earth
Sacral	Water
Solar Plexus	Fire
Heart	Air
Throat	Akasa
Brow	None
Crown	None

Each of the chakras is assigned to a ruling deity or pair of deities. These figures act as initiators into the essential experience of the chakra. The deities are often depicted with many heads and arms to indicate their various qualities or aspects. The god-forms hold items that symbolise the lessons that the chakra holds for the aspirant. These symbols can be used as focal points in meditation. When the student has an understanding of these symbols, the deities can be visualised holding all the various items.

The dual rulership of each chakra, except in the case of the brow chakra, is especially interesting. The chakras are constantly moderating yin and yang energies. The point of balance is personified by the male and female deities. The deity representing the ajna (brow) chakra is androgynous: both male and female. It is at this point that the ida and pingala currents merge with sushumna to create one current which is neither yin nor yang.

The deities make two gestures, the abhayamudra to dispel fears and the varada to grant boons. If the chakra is approached in the right spirit there is nothing to fear. If you wish to work with the eastern deities you will need to study the relevant mythologies and understand the forces they represent, and you will need to be able to visualise their forms clearly. If you are unable to do this, visualise a pair of rulers for each chakra, perhaps as lord and lady or even as king and queen. Use an androgynous figure for the ajna chakra.

The Chakras: Presiding Deities

CHAKRA	DEITIES
Base	Brahma holding staff, gourd, rosary
	Dakini holding spear, staff with skull atop, sword, cup
Sacral	Vishnu holding conch shell, disc, war club, lotus
	Rakini holding trident, lotus, drum, battle axe
Solar Plexus	Rudra holding rosary, fire weapon
	Lakini holding thunderbolt, fire weapon
Heart	Isa holds nothing
	Kakini holding noose, skull
Throat	Sadasiva holding noose, goad, serpent, trident, fire weapon, vajra, sword, battle axe, sword, bell
	Gauri holding noose, goad, arrow, bow
Brow	Sakti Hakini holding book, drum, staff with skull, rosary

Visualisation is not an exercise in mental skill. It is the creation of an appropriate vehicle, a thought form. The act of visualising draws upon the faculties of the right hemisphere of the brain, which also provides the ability to understand symbolic forms. Drawing upon this hemisphere also calls into play emotional depths that remain untapped by sheer rationalisation. Building a god-form in the mind's eye should elicit an emotional reaction. If it does not, the exercise is not being performed to the fullest. The Tibetan tradition includes highly complex and detailed visualisation of deities. These are invariably dissolved into emptiness at the termination of the practice.

The functions of the chakras are additionally symbolised by various animals. These are the elephant with seven trunks, the makara—a crocodile-like creature—the ram and the antelope. These also have mythological connections with certain deities. The elephant with seven trunks is Airavata, the elephant of Indra. At the base chakra Airavata wears a black collar to indicate that he is bound to the forces of ignorance. This chakra is assigned to the element of earth. The elephant reappears without the restrictive black noose as the symbol for the throat chakra. The elephant is now pure white indicating freedom from ignorance. The makara, symbol of the svadisthana chakra (assigned to water), is the emblem of Varuna, lord of the seas. The ram found at the solar plexus chakra (assigned to fire) is the companion to Agni, the god of fire. The gazelle or antelope, found at the heart chakra (assigned to air) is the vehicle of Vayu god of the winds. These animal symbols underline the elemental correspondences and also carry the mantra for each chakra.

The mantra is a sounded meditation that resonates with the vibration of the chakra. Each chakra is assigned to a different bija mantra or seed syllable. Starting at the base chakra the bija mantras are Lam, Vam, Ram, Yam, Ham and Om. There is no bija mantra for the crown chakra. Each of these seed sounds is depicted within the centre of the lotus. The *Sat-Cakra-Nirupana* describes these mantras as being seated upon the back of the appropriate animal. In effect, the text presents us with a powerful constellation of related images. The mantra rides upon the animal, set within the yantra, watched by the deities bearing symbolic gifts. These are all encompassed within the circle, set about with petals inscribed with Sanskrit letters. Here are the keys to the chakras, they await you.

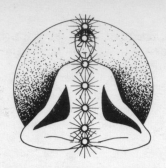

4 · THE GATEWAY OF EARTH

THE BASE CHAKRA: TABLE OF CORRESPONDENCES

Location Perineum, between the anus and the genitals
Sanskrit name Muladhara, derived from mula meaning 'root' and 'adhara' meaning base or support
Function Survival, grounding
Element Earth
Inner State Stability
Glands Adrenals
Body parts Legs, feet, bones, large intestine
Malfunction Obesity, haemorrhoids, constipation, sciatica
Colour Red
Seed sound Lam
Sense Smell
Vowel sound O as in rope
Petals Four: vam, śaṃ, ṣam, saṃ
Animal symbols Bull, elephant, ox
Deities Brahma, Dakini
  Gaia, Demeter, Persephone, Erishkagel, Ana, Ceres, Ceridwen, Geb, Hades, Pwyll

GOD: *Child Brahma*   GODDESS: *Dakini*

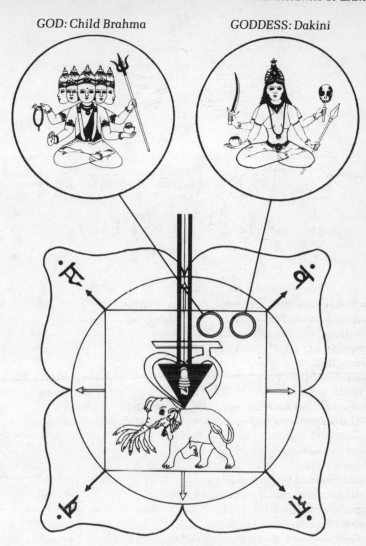

Muladhara Chakra
From *Kundalini Yoga for the West*

By meditating thus on Her who shines within the Mula-Cakra, with the lustre of ten million Suns, a man becomes Lord of Speech, and a King among men and an adept in all kinds of learning.

Sat-Cakra-Nirupana, verse 13

Our journey begins here at the base chakra. The Sanskrit name for this chakra is muladhara. It is drawn from two words meaning 'root' and 'base' or 'support'. This aptly describes the function of this centre, namely to provide a powerful anchor that links us with all living things. It is our base in the physical world. We too are part of nature; we share many functions and instincts with other living creatures; we are all part of one world. If we fail to acknowledge such things we are simply deluded. This sense of belonging within the physical world is vital in our dealings with it. If we believe ourselves to be separate from the natural world as outsiders, observers and manipulators we make a grave and deadly error.

The base chakra primarily represents the will to survive, the fundamental drive itself. Without this drive there is no willingness to battle against adverse circumstances or to adapt to new situations. Animals also express the will to survive through their own evolutionary development.

It is ironic that precisely this collective skill at survival now threatens the well-being and possibly survival of the Earth herself. The current reappearance of the shamanistic path is a significant development at this time of crisis. The shaman is essentially a tribal figure, a walker in two worlds, magician, healer and source of practical wisdom. It is a path which is rooted in the land and the natural world. Animal totems clearly link man and the kingdoms of nature into a unified whole. The vision-quest, an essential experience upon the shamanistic path, is a spiritual quest which is rooted in the physical world and the skills of survival. It is a test not just of the individual's ability to communicate with the unseen forces of the higher worlds but it is also a test of survival in the natural world. The wilderness initiation is making a much-needed reappearance as part of a general move to rediscover spiritual values in the land and the environment. Here lies a true grounding experience which reveals the unity between humanity and nature. If we cannot perceive spiritual meaning in the world about us, there is little point in looking for it in the abstract and the intangible.

The colour red is attributed to this chakra. It is the colour of life blood. Red ochre was frequently smeared on the bodies of the dead to represent rebirth into a new life. It has come to symbolise the passions and the life force itself. The colour has passed into common usage in the language: when we are angry we see red; if we paint the town red, we indulge in extravagant and boisterous behaviour. The colour red is assigned to the planet Mars, which symbolises dynamic, energetic and even aggressive forces. The colour red exhibits the lowest frequency in the colour spectrum. It corresponds well to the qualities and functions of the base chakra.

The base chakra, unlike the others, faces downwards towards the earth where it picks up and transmits subtle geodetic forces. Such contact is dependent upon proximity to the physical earth. The trappings of civilisation can insulate us totally unless we make a conscious effort to counterbalance this effect. Walking in an open place is not just good exercise, it is a good opportunity to connect with the earth beneath our feet.

The base chakra is well named. It represents our most primitive instincts and drives. It is not surprising that the glands associated with this chakra are the adrenals, which are responsible for the fight or flight response through the output of adrenalin. This is a primitive response, a leftover from those distant days when our ancestors had to run or fight for their lives. We like to think of ourselves as being civilised and sophisticated, but in dire situations we can find ourselves battling for daily survival, as did our forefathers.

The word 'mula' means root. Swami Satyananda Saraswati, a modern teacher and founder of the Bihar school of Yoga, reminds us that 'mula' is best understood as mula-prakriti, the transcendental basis of all natural phenomena, the origin to which matter again returns upon disintegration. We now know that a strange subatomic world of particles underpins our own world of physical manifestation. Here is the stuff of mountains, seas and plains, the root of stars and planets. Yet to the outer senses this world is invisible and inaccessible. It obeys a different set of rules from those which govern the physical world. Nevertheless our roots emerge from this foreign domain, energy miraculously becomes matter. The subatomic world is still a place of great mystery, only gradually yielding its secrets.

The transformative power, Kundalini, is also a great mystery. We cannot study the chakras without considering it any more than we can look at seven colours without realising that they form a rainbow. This dormant power rests within the base chakra. The complete rising of this force is said to bring liberation and enlightenment. When the power is awakened, it rises up through the chakras and transforms all in its path.

The traditional Hindu symbols depict the qualities and functions of this chakra. Accordingly this chakra has four petals. The sephirah Malkuth, which corresponds to the base chakra, is also subdivided into four parts to symbolise the four elements. The four petals of this chakra are each inscribed with the Sanskrit letters Vam, Sam, Sam, Sam in gold. Within the circumference of the chakra is a yellow square, privithi, the yantra of earth. Privithi means 'the wide earth' and is revered as a goddess. Among her children are the dawn, fire and the god Indra. Privithi represents the stability of physical manifestation. Once again there is a parallel with the western tradition which also symbolises the stability of material forms with a square. There is an arrow at each of the corners and also at the midway points. These represent directions or possibilities which are ever open to the individual at the physical level. There is always a danger of dispersing energies by chasing too many goals at one time. Discrimination has to be developed in order to focus the mind. Within the square there is a white elephant with seven trunks. This is Airavata, the elephant of Indra. Satyananda tells us that the seven trunks represent the seven minerals necessary for physical life. The elephant has been both warrior and worker in India. It is renowned for its strength and intelligence. It has also come to symbolise the mind which, without training, is wild and potentially destructive. The elephant is also found in the fifth chakra to indicate that the mental powers have been trained and put into service.

Traditionally each chakra is ruled by a divine pair. Here we find Brahma depicted as a child with his consort Dakini. The child nature of the god-form indicates the relative immaturity of consciousness at this level. The deities each bear a number of items which symbolise the lessons that the base chakra has to teach. Brahma carries a danda or staff, a gourd and a rosary. He makes a gesture which dispels fear. The staff represents the spine as the outer form of the channel through which Kundalini can rise. The gourd is often used as a drinking cup and represents the slaking of spiritual thirst. The rosary has 108 beads which represent the many names of the Divine Mother, the Shakti of manifestation.

Dakini carries a spear, a sword, a staff with a skull at the top and a cup. She too makes a gesture to dispel fear. The spear represents the need to achieve our own targets, the sword represents the power of discrimination, the staff symbolises the empty mind and the cup represents the waters of life from which the aspirant hopes to drink. It is almost impossible not to be reminded of certain western elemental symbols: the cup, sword, the staff and spear.

Within the square just above the symbol of the elephant we see a trikona, a triangle pointing downwards. This represents Shakti, the feminine aspect of creation. In the western tradition a downward pointing triangle stands for the element of water which is also considered to be female in polarity. The trikona contains the Shiva lingam—the phallus—around which a serpent is coiled three and a half times. This is the sleeping Kundalini force which makes three and a half circuits to complete its upward journey. Above the phallus is a small crescent moon—a citkala—symbol of the divine source of all energy.

Here we have some profound teachings about the universal nature of polarity, the union of opposites in ceaseless momentum. The Shiva–Shakti polarity is but one manifestation of the sacred marriage, the union which brings the irreconcilable opposites together. Shakti, the feminine force, is assigned to the base chakra. Shiva, the masculine force, is assigned to the crown. We are being presented with the irresistible magnetism between matter and spirit. When the two are separated a state of duality prevails. Without this separation manifestation could not take place. When Kundalini rises fully, Shiva and Shakti unite. Cosmic consciousness is born from their union.

There is a particular polarity between this chakra and that of the crown. The base chakra holds the root of Kundalini; the crown chakra, 'the abode of Shiva', opens fully at the ultimate flowering. Kundalini as Shakti resides at the base chakra awaiting the future cosmic union. Matters of personal sexuality belong more properly to the second chakra. Here is the universal law, the attraction of opposites which underlies creation. The Shiva–Shakti polarity is a paradigm of creation itself. In this axis we can seen the great cosmic forces particularised and personalised.

Hindu metaphysics portrays manifestation as a series of emanations producing increasingly dense levels of existence. All aspects of the creative force are essentially masculine–feminine partnerships embodying active and passive principles. To underline this conception Hindu deities are often paired, gods and goddesses with the same root name but distinguished by different endings to emphasise their qualities: Isvara, Isvari and Brahma, Brahmini for example. The term Shakti refers to the feminine aspect at all levels of creation. When it is added to the name of a goddess it reinforces her nature as a dynamic co-creator at a certain level. There is a hierarchy of Shakti powers symbolised as active partners within the chakras themselves. The Divine Feminine has dominion over the matter of the material world providing form as a container for force. Kundalini Shakti, resident at the base chakra, is a cosmic force omnipresent throughout creation. It is particularised within a human being. Kundalini eventually rises at the behest of consciousness that has been awakened through spiritual practice.

The sahasrara-muladhara axis can be visualised as a magnetic force with an attractive pole at each end. Separating the two poles of the magnet are a number of blockages, obstacles or knots which prevent the transmission of magnetic force. Spiritual practice has the effect of removing such obstacles. When there is nothing standing between the two opposite but mutually attracting poles a reaction takes place. The earth pole itself undergoes transformation, after which it no longer has dominion. Instead, the ruling powers are transferred to the crown, transcendent spiritual reality. The powers of the muladhara chakra rise in a transformed state and unite with the powers of the sahasrara chakra. From this union of opposites transcendent consciousness is born. This image, though mechanistic and contrived, helps us to imagine the unimaginable and to envisage what we are unlikely to experience for ourselves.

Hindu teachings tell us that the base chakra itself contains a psychic knot, the brahma granthi. These are also found at the heart and brow chakras. These 'knots' have to be dissolved at their respective points to allow the evolutionary energies to flow upwards. These psychic blocks cannot be taken by force nor dismantled by the intellect. This can only be accomplished through an inner shift in orientation which releases the grip of the ego and dissolves the illusions relevant at each level. The existence of these knots within the energy centres acts as a most important safeguard contributing to the maintenance of the status quo. They act as closed doors which inhibit the rising of energy beyond certain levels until consciousness itself has created the necessary key.

In the body this chakra rules the legs and feet, the bones and the large intestines. Imbalances at this level can bring about obesity, sciatica, haemorrhoids, constipation and, in men, prostate problems. Individuals with these difficulties would benefit from working with the energies of the base chakra. Imbalances at this level can also create psychological problems such as conditions of grief, depression and instability. These reflect darkened views of the world. Self-indulgent behaviour such as greed, avarice and extreme self-centredness, which each represent limited views about the self, can also result from blockages at this level. Over-identification with this state of consciousness brings an excessive concern for material stability and external values such as status, power and prestige. The restricted outlook then becomes self-perpetuating. It is not difficult to see this kind of consciousness in the world at large.

The base chakra houses karmic forces. Chakras hold information and memory like computer discs constantly updating the amount of life data on file. The contents of each chakra remain undisclosed until the appropriate 'key' is recognised. This key can take many forms, for example applied energy, meditation or physical stimulus. A sudden awakening can unexpectedly tap distant memory and release repressed emotions in a volcanic way.

When the base chakra is active and balanced there is a sense of purpose, a sense of belonging to the natural world and a willingness to take personal responsibility for actions and deeds.

ORIENTATION EXERCISES

1. Choose an earth deity. Study their mythology and familiarise yourself with the forms in which they have been represented.
2. Explore your own relationship with the natural world by considering: What does the earth give you and what do you give the earth?
3. Meditate on the element of earth.

ASANAS

1. BODY DROPS

This exercise works on governor vessel 1 at the base of the spine.
1. Sit on the floor with legs stretched out in front of you.
2. Support yourself by placing your hands on the floor behind you.
3. Arch your buttocks and bounce gently on the base of the spine.

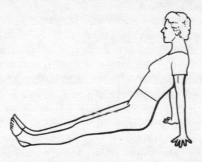

Body drops

2. LEG STRETCHES

This exercise stretches the sciatic nerve, which is the largest nerve in the body.

1. Sit on the floor with legs outstretched in front of you.
2. Lift upwards in the spine
3. Bend your right knee and place the heel between the genitals and rectum, so that you are sitting on the heel. This stimulates conception vessel 1. Your left leg remains straight out in front.
4. Reach forward and take hold of your leg at the shin, ankle or even the foot if this is comfortable.
5. Exhale and bend forwards, bring your head towards the left knee, but do not slump the spine forwards.
6. Repeat by working on the other side of the body.

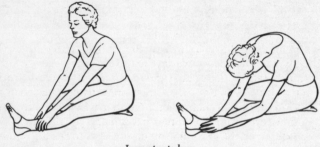

Leg stretches

3. SITTING ON THE HEELS (VAJRASANA)

Sitting in Vajrasana stimulates the urinary meridian which runs down the back of the legs. Concentrating on the nose stimulates the muladhara by focusing on the point where ida and pingala terminate. Concentrating the perineum focuses awareness on the area where ida and pingala originate.

1. Sit on the heels with the knees pointing forwards and slightly apart.
2. Interlock the hands and hold them below the navel with wrists on the thighs.
3. Close the eyes and direct the attention to the tip of your nose for several minutes as a meditation.
4. Shift the attention to the perineum for several minutes as a meditation. The perineum can also be contracted and relaxed sequentially.

VISUALISATION: THE FOUR HORIZONS

See before you a circle traced out upon the ground. See the four directions marked clearly on it. In the centre of the circle stands a figure wearing a dark robe of coarse cloth with a hood. This is your chosen earth deity. As you watch, the figure invites you to stand in the centre of the circle. You stand together at the centre. The figure draws a small rod from the folds of the cloak and points towards the distant eastern horizon.

You find yourself watching a group of men hunting together on foot armed only with spears and sticks. Now you run beside them as they pursue a great animal ahead. They surround the great beast, which towers over them. They work together, attacking and wounding the giant creature to bring it down. You feel something of their experience: terror mingled with excitement, exuberance combined with concentration. You feel a flush of adrenalin. As the beast is brought down, your legs seem to give way as if you too had participated in the chase and the kill.

The scene fades and you return to the centre of the circle. The figure directs your attention towards the next horizon. Now you find yourself amidst great clouds of dust and the sound of the clash of arms. You are in the thick of battle. Two armies are pitting themselves one against the other, without mercy. You wonder why they have taken to arms. You hear the sound of horses in pain and the distant cries of men cut and dying on the ground. You do not wait to see the outcome of the day for you cannot know if the victor has a just cause. You can only see the slaughter of men and hear the sounds of battle. You turn away. The scene fades and you return to the central point.

Your guide directs your attention to the next quarter. Find yourself standing at a city gate. A steep cobbled street rises ahead. On either side of the street people lie, or sit hunched up, motionless. Ragged children hang on to emaciated women. At the top of the rise the street opens out onto a square, which is decorated with flags and regalia. Yet in the doorways and corners around the square you can still see the ragged figures. Into the square comes a great procession: soldiers, musicians and dancers all in extravagant costumes. Now come the rulers of the city, carried aloft in decorated palanquins by men. They pass in a blaze of colour. You turn away. The scene fades. You are back at the central point again.

Your guide directs your attention to the last quarter. You find yourself transported to a small hillside overlooking a paddy field. In the field a group of women are at work planting rice. They are bent over as they work. You watch them as they work, slowly, patiently, methodically moving through the field in a subtle rhythm of work. You hope that their harvest will be a good one. The whole community depends upon it. The scene fades from view and you find yourself standing at the central point once more.

Beside you is the figure of your chosen deity. The figure turns to you and speaks: 'You have watched others; how will you use the powers of earth?' Take time to reflect. The scene finally fades.

DREAM IMAGES

Work on the base chakra can spontaneously produce a wide range of images, indicating that an awakening has taken place, for example dreams that take place underground and reveal a hitherto untapped source of power, possibly in a subterranean chamber, basement or cellar; dreams of underground fire; dreams of opening a hidden trap door; dreams that feature digging for hidden treasure or unearthing items of significance. Dreams featuring a serpent, bull, elephant or other massive beast also relate to this level of consciousness.

BACH FLOWER REMEDIES

Cherry plum	6	Learning to let go
Clematis	9	Grounding
Gorse	13	Integration of joy and sorrow
Pine	24	Taking responsibility for your own life
Sweet chestnut	30	Trusting your own development

MUSIC

This chakra responds to earthy tribal music and primitive natural rhythms. The authentic sounds of drumming or chanting may encourage you to dance, stamp your feet or jump. Suggested pieces are *Meetings with Remarkable Alloys* by Chris Campell or *Spirit of The Red Man* by John Richardson.

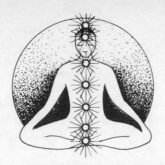

5 · THE GATEWAY OF THE MOON

THE SACRAL CHAKRA: TABLE OF
CORRESPONDENCES

Location The sacral plexus

Sanskrit name Svadisthana, meaning 'sweetness', or 'one's own abode'

Element Water

Function Pleasure, sexuality, procreation, creativity

Inner state Self-confidence, well-being

Body parts Womb, kidneys, reproductive system, circulation system, bladder

Glands Ovaries, Testicles

Malfunction Impotence, frigidity, uterine, bladder or kidney trouble

Colour Orange

Seed sound Vam

Sense Taste

Petals Six: bam, bham, mam, yam, ram, lam

Animal symbols Makara, fish, sea creatures

Deities Vishnu, Rakini

He who meditates upon this stainless Lotus, which is named Svadisthana, is freed immediately from all his enemies.

Sat-Cakra-Nirupana, verse 18

GOD: *Visnu*   GODDESS: *Sakti Rakini*

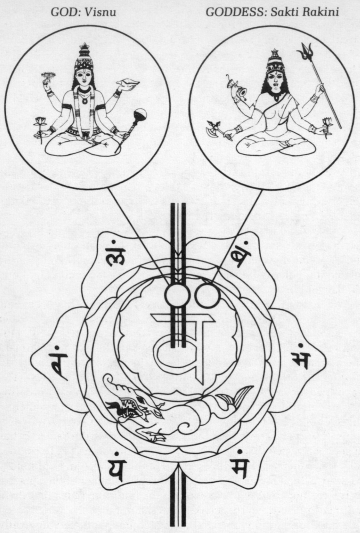

Svadhisthana Chakra
From Kundalini Yoga for the West

Rising up from the base chakra, we now encounter the second chakra, svadisthana. The roots of the muladhara and svadisthana chakras are located close together so that some functions are shared. This chakra is related to the sacral nerve plexus.

There is some debate about the derivation of the name. Some authorities translate it to mean 'sweetness'. Svadisthana is after all the centre for physical pleasure. Others believe that the word is derived from sva meaning 'that which belongs to itself' and dhisthana meaning 'its actual place'. It therefore means 'one's own abode'. It has been suggested that this refers to a distant time when Kundalini lay dormant within the sacral chakra.

This chakra is located within the abdomen, midway between the pubis and the navel. It governs sexuality, procreation and creativity at all levels. Physically this chakra affects the flow of fluids in the body. Its element, not surprisingly, is water.

The major function of this chakra is procreation and sexuality, and in fact it is inactive until puberty. Sexuality is the prime manifestation of the attraction between opposites. The yin yang symbol expresses the fundamental polarity between opposites: male and female, light and dark, day and night, sun and moon.

In the human family sexuality and procreation have become separated through the evolution of menstruation over oestrus. Neither procreation nor sexual activity is limited to a short season. This evolutionary step has been a vital factor in the social development of the human family. Theo Lang writes of the important link between the human sex drive and the socialising results when he says, 'The year-round sexual urge can therefore be seen as the dominating factor in forming human society.'[1] Sexuality takes on a social as well as a biological function and tends to produce patterns of social organisation that permit long-term bonding across the sexes. It has also been suggested that the continuous activity of the sex hormones results in an increased alertness in the brain and also in exploratory behaviour, which favour the successful establishment of the species. This interesting point tends to confirm the traditional idea that there is a direct link between this chakra and the mind.

The function of human sexuality is complex, both sociologically and psychologically. It has opened human development to the possibility of intimate relationships. However, the power structures that have been created to control sexuality have often produced the ugliest defilement and persecution of women. The perennial issues concerning the use and abuse of sexual power face every generation and indeed every individual.

There is doubtless a difference between the ways in which men and women experience sexuality. This is a direct reflection of different energy patterns, quite apart from biological differences and social conditioning. In women the second chakra includes the womb, and the chakra can be seen emanating from within the body. It gives rise to a sexuality that is usually deeply felt and experienced within the wholeness of being. A man lacks the womb as a deep anchor point and often sexual experiences remain emotionally unconnected. In men the second chakra is sometimes integrated but it can also be seen as a sphere hovering outside the body. This is not to deny that men are capable of deep sexual experience, but such experience follows integration and is dependent upon it. The trigger for the process of integration can take many forms. It can be self-initiated or it can begin when a man finds a partner who awakens the anima within. It may never take place at all, giving rise to the hunting male, ever-hungry for sexual conquest, who will never find more than ego satisfaction.

Sexuality is an area that is now bearing the full weight of the ongoing battles between the sexes. In society this manifests in many contending issues. Sexual behaviour has undergone a recent revolution, in the west at least. This revision of attitudes and morality brings us face to face with the very nature of sexuality and its purpose in our lives.

Sexuality and spirituality are usually considered to be worlds apart. Those who enter the spiritual life as monks, priests or nuns give up a sex life and become celibate choosing instead to channel the emotions through a life of service. Celibacy is inextricably bound to the religious values of the tradition itself. In the past some faiths, notably Christianity, promulgated celibacy as a means of overcoming the so-called temptations of the flesh. This attitude has left its legacy. Sex can still be thought of as a defilement of spiritual purity. The sex drive becomes the enemy within; it must be defeated at all cost. The practices that developed to keep the second chakra under control remain punitive, dour and repressive.

By contrast, it is possible to follow the path of celibacy by transmuting the sex drive rather than seeking to destroy it. This is a more positive and accepting approach. The life energies that are generated through the second chakra circulate upwards into the higher chakras, like a rising head of steam. Sexuality is transmuted; the energies that would have been available for a personal relationship are now freed from that constraint and become available on a far wider basis. Life energies can flow to the many, not merely to the one.

The sexual energies can be aligned to the higher centres, especially to the fifth centre. The Tibetan states that when the energies of the sacral centre 'are reorientated and carried up to the throat centre, then the aspirant becomes a conscious creative force in the higher worlds. He (she) enters within the veil and begins to create the pattern of things which will bring about eventually the new heavens and the new earth.[2]

There is a natural polarity between the forces of the second chakra and those of the fifth which appears in the Qabalah. Yesod symbolises the second chakra, Daath symbolises the fifth chakra. Daath is often described as Yesod upon a higher arc. This polarity works to transmute the forces of physical creation into genuine creativity.

Sexual activity itself can be transformative. The intensity of sexual encounter can awaken higher centres and transcend the physical confines of the experience. In the past such avenues have been explored as ways of unifying the split between body and spirit, sexuality and spirituality. Sexual alchemy expresses personal transformation through sexual union. This approach to sexuality is quite different from the instinct-dominated drive. It requires a high degree of mental control, physical discipline and absolute equality across the sexes.

In the Tantric tradition sexuality is elevated to a sacramental status. The personal sexual union symbolises the cosmic union, the meeting of male and female polarities. Sex can become a means of liberating personal energy from the narrow confines of social conditioning and personal desire. The raw power of personal passion becomes the fuel for transforming personal consciousness into transcendence. The energies of the second chakra are consciously raised towards the highest source imaginable.

When we look at the traditional chakra images themselves we can discover more about the functions of this centre. The svadisthana chakra has six petals, which are coloured vermilion. This bright, strong colour indicates that the impulses, ideas and desires generated here are stimulating to the mind. The creative artist ever in search of the face of the Muse stands as living proof to this. A sexual relationship can become the wellspring for truly inspired creativity.

The yantra for this chakra is a crescent moon. Its animal symbol is a makara, an alligator-like creature, the Leviathan of the waters, according to Jung. The element assigned to this chakra is water. In sharp contrast to the element of earth which is fixed and immobile, water has no shape of its own but takes on a shape from the surroundings. Water can be deceptive, calm upon the surface but turbulent and dangerous beneath. It has a reflective surface quality, almost like a mirror. There is a natural affinity between the waters and the moon, which exerts a powerful tidal influence. All life begins in waters of the womb. We all share this experience but do not remember. The element of water symbolises our shared ancestral past, the collective mind, ever-present yet beyond the realm of memory.

Water carries a deeply symbolic value within many major spiritual traditions. It symbolises purification, the washing away of imperfection. Ritual bathing or washing is a universal practice as a preparation for spiritual observance. Baptism through full or partial immersion into sanctified water is a widespread practice which marks the entry into the religious life. It represents birth consciously undertaken. Holy water is often thought to have special powers. Ancient Egyptian temples inevitably included a sacred lake which symbolised the primal waters from which the first mound, the Benben arose. Ceremonial creation dramas were enacted on and around the lake at special times. The Christian creation story also includes the image of the waters: 'The Spirit of God moved upon the face of the waters.'

Water is a powerful symbol. It is not surprising that it appears in all traditions and it expresses universal truths which we each understand at a deep level of our being.

In the western tradition this chakra is represented by Yesod. It is assigned both lunar and water symbols. The moon is attributed to Yesod. Its forever hidden face is a powerful symbol of the collective unconscious and the hidden depths of the subconscious mind. Yesod also signifies the astral level, a level of reality created by massed thought forms and charged emotions. The astral world and the collective unconscious are essentially shared yet hidden forces. Perhaps the former is an active expression of the latter. Both are equally well symbolised as a great sea. The fish or sea creature is a classic symbol for contacting the deep and turbulent waters of the subconscious or for interacting with the astral world. Riding upon the back of a turtle, playing with dolphins and meeting mermaids each refer to this contact. Such images appear in dreams and within the collective storehouse of legends and myths.

It is interesting to discover that lunar symbolism is found in both eastern and western systems as a means of describing this chakra. The moon is identified with the hidden unconscious forces; one face is always hidden from us. Lunar symbols by tradition have been identified with women whose menstrual rhythms also follow a cyclic pattern. The moon is connected with all waters: the rise of sap, the flow of blood and the movement of the tides. It is these waters that appear in our dreams as living symbols of inner states: the gushing fountains, the great sea, the dank pool, the dried up river bed or the frozen wastes. These images inform us of our own inner world that we have created from our thoughts which in turn have arisen from our desires.

In the body the second chakra governs all liquids: the circulation of blood, the production of urine, menstrual flow and the production of seminal fluids. Blockages or imbalances can cause disruption in any of these systems. This chakra is also connected with the kidney, bladder and triple heater meridians. The svadisthana chakra also has a profound bearing on certain states of mind. If the chakra is overly yang there can be undue emphasis on sexual activity joined to excessive fantasy. If the chakra is overly yin impotence or other sexual problems can appear. Frustration both sexual and creative can be generated here when the life energies are blocked.

The presiding deities are Vishnu and Rakini, an aspect of Sarasvati. Sarasvati is an ancient river goddess who is identified with speech and eloquence which is, after all, a flow of words. She is the mother of the Vedas and rides upon a swan or sits on a lotus. Visnu is regarded as being one of the most important of the gods. He may take many forms, including that of a fish.

Vishnu wears a garland of forest flowers from all seasons, the vanamala. He carries a conch, a disc, a mace and a lotus. The conch symbolises the need to develop attentive listening; it also provides a link with the element of water. The disc tells us that concentration is required if we are to hit our target. The mace or war club reminds us of the need to subdue the ego, and the lotus reminds us of the spiritual goal itself.

The goddess Rakini carries a trident, a drum, a lotus and a battle axe. She has a fierce face with protruding teeth to remind us of the dangers of the untrained imagination. Her trident is a symbol of the essential unity of mind, body and spirit. It is reminiscent of the trident carried by Poseidon, the Greek god of the seas. The drum beats out the rhythm of life. The battle axe symbolises the struggle which the aspirant faces to overcome the negative aspects of self. The lotus reminds us of the victory that is possible for everyone.

The seed sound for this chakra is vam. The syllables inscribed upon the six petals are lam, ram, yam, mam, bam and bham.

When this chakra awakens it brings increased powers of intuition and increasing psychic abilities. It is also said to bring awareness of the astral form. Awakening this chakra can affect the sex drive dramatically, either positively or negatively. In each case the effects are usually short-lived and stabilise as the energies settle. During the phase of awakening it is not uncommon to become oversensitive to every external stimulus. Hiroshi Motoyama reports that during this phase his emotions became unstable and he was easily excited. During meditation even the smallest noise sounded like thunder. I myself also experienced a considerable degree of instability. I felt as though my external protective layer had been stripped away; I could not sleep or rest until exhausted; every sense was sharpened to a painful degree. I was overwhelmed by the karmic pressures that were released.

The karmic forces at this level belong to the collective unconscious. These are the forces and experiences that have shaped the evolution of our race. Individual far memories will be stored as part of this great pool. This chakra can release a karmic deluge which can prove insurmountable to Kundalini rising from muladhara. The svadisthana chakra has to be cleared of karmic debris before Kundalini can rise any higher.

When this chakra is balanced it brings a sense of self-confidence and creativity. The imagination is used constructively and sexual energy brings a sense of completeness and integration.

ORIENTATION EXERCISES

1. How do you use the function of sexuality? What meaning does it have for you?
2. Meditate on the element of water.

ASANAS

1. THE LOCUST POSE (SHALHALABASANA)

1. Lie on your stomach with your hands beside your thighs with palms down.
2. Stretch and raise your legs with your abdomen as high as possible keeping the knees straight. Hold for a few seconds and then lower to the floor.
Repeat up to five times.

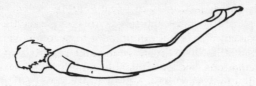

The Locust Pose

2. THE CAT–COW POSE

1. Place your hands and knees on the floor. so that you are making a bridge with your back.
2. Inhale, arch the back and raise your head.
3. Exhale, round the back and drop the head downwards. Establish a rhythm of inhaling, head up and exhaling, head down. Continue this for about one minute.

This exercise works on points along the spine including governor vessels 3, 4 and 5. These points are called the Gates of Life.

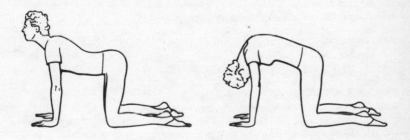

The Cat–Cow Pose

3. LEG-LIFTS

1. Lie on your back and relax.
2. Lift your legs about six inches away from the floor.

3. Spread them apart a little, bring the legs together and then kick out.

VISUALISATION: THE WOMB OF THE MOTHER

Darkness surrounds you, yet the dark feels comforting and safe. You are floating suspended in water. You are immersed in water, surrounded and held by water. You feel safe here, floating in these warm waters. You are in the womb, deep in the womb of the one who nurtured you. You are surrounded by her body, held in her waters. You move and sway floating in your bubble. Here there are no thoughts, no fears, just life, growing, changing, developing. Life grows within the waters, quietly unfolding according to the pattern. You are surrounded by another's life, beyond the waters. This great being surrounds you with her love. You cannot name this feeling, nor understand it. But you grow in its presence as time passes. You feel safe, surrounded by love, immersed in love, floating in the waters. Time has no meaning for you but time passes and the waters change.

You know the waters in a deep primal sense, as you know no other element. You grew and were nourished by the waters. You floated in the waters while nine moons passed. You filled the waters and were finally born from them. You have no conscious memory of that time spent in the darkness of the waters, yet your consciousness can remember the feelings of that blissful state. Every human being has passed this way too. Every human being begins in the darkness and the waters. There is no other way into life.

DREAM IMAGES

This chakra tends to produce dreams in which water images appear: images of pools, lakes, streams, rivers and seas. The quality of the water is indicative of the way in which this chakra is functioning. Stagnant, dirty or foul water requires inner cleansing. Frozen water, ice in any form requires thawing. Images of bathing or washing are indicative that a cleansing process has commenced. Swimming indicates ease with the functions of this chakra. Drowning indicates difficulties. Fountains or gushing waters indicate the sudden or unexpected awaking of this chakra. Meetings with creatures or beings who are at home in the waters and are willing to act as guides indicate that the individual is integrating some aspect of this chakra.

Dreams in which the moon plays a prominent part are also related to this chakra; travelling to the moon or exploring a lunar landscape indicate inner exploration at this level. Meeting figures or guides who mediate a lunar force also represents inner work in this area.

Bach Flower Remedies

Crab apple	10	Getting rid of what you cannot digest
Elm	11	Turning your ideas into reality
Mimulus	20	Freedom within a structure
Oak	22	Surrender
Vervain	31	Accepting others
Wild rose	37	Taking part joyfully in life

Music

Sensual flowing music is appropriate here. Listen to traditional music for belly dancing. This has the power to release the energies of this chakra.

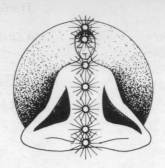

6 · THE GATEWAY OF THE SUN

THE SOLAR PLEXUS CHAKRA: TABLE OF
CORRESPONDENCES.

Location Rooted between the twelfth thoracic vertebra and first
lumbar vertebra
Sanskrit name Manipura, meaning 'lustrous gem' or 'city of jewels'
Element Fire
Function Will, power
Inner state Intense emotion: laughter, joy, anger
Body parts Digestive system, liver, spleen, stomach, small intestine
Glands Pancreas
Malfunction Ulcers, diabetes, eating disorders such as anorexia and
bulimia, hypoglycaemia
Colour Yellow
Seed sound Ram
Sense Sight
Petals Ten: da, dha, na, ta, tha, da, dha, na, pa, pha
Animal symbols Ram
Deities Rudra, Lakini
  Apollo, Agni

By meditating on this navel lotus, the power to destroy and create is acquired.
Sat-Cakra-Nirupana, verse 21

We rise up from the fluid svadisthana chakra to encounter the fire
of the manipura chakra. Satyananda locates this chakra between the

GOD: Visnu   GODDESS: Lakini

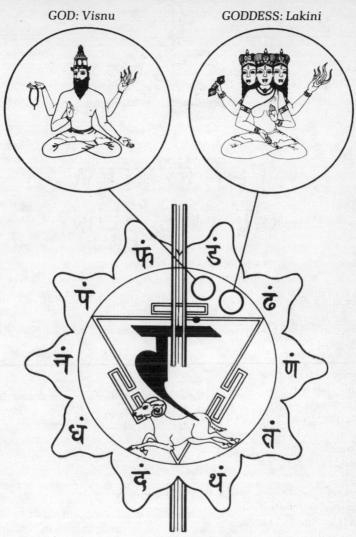

Manipura Chakra
From Kundalini Yoga for the West

twelfth thoracic vertebra and the first lumbar vertebra behind the navel. In the west this chakra is known as the solar plexus chakra. This is something of a misnomer as the twelve thoracic nerves in this area do not form a plexus but remain separate.

Manipura can be translated as 'lustrous gem', 'city of jewels' or 'filled with jewels'. In Tibet this chakra is known as manipadma or 'jewelled lotus'. This chakra radiates its fiery energy like a bright sun. Its colour is yellow, its element is fire.

The abdomen contains the digestive system which transmutes food into energy. We rarely think about this process, except when it malfunctions in some way. Food provides fuel for the body. Just as the physical digestive system extracts energy from food, so the solar plexus chakra extracts and stores prana.

Prana is the energy that permeates all life; where there is prana there is life. Each of the chakras is a centre of prana, but it is generated and distributed by the manipura centre. Prana can be directed to any of the body's systems through the power of the directed imagination in conjunction with a sound knowledge of anatomy.

Prana Vidya is the practical study of the life force. This is an ancient branch of esoteric training originating in the Tantric tradition. Practitioners are taught the techniques of contraction, expansion and localisation of prana. Disturbances of prana in the body are considered to be the root cause of disease. Prana can be directed from one person to another especially during a healing encounter. It can sometimes be seen as brilliant flashes of white light emanating from the hands. During an energy exchange sudden changes in temperature are often experienced, depending upon the direction of the flow. The healer, the one directing prana, often experiences the sensation of heat followed by extreme coldness as prana is first built up and then released. The one receiving prana often experiences a gradual warming sensation as prana is slowly assimilated.

In the body, prana is traditionally said to have five forms or winds called udana, samana, uyana, apana and prana. Udana governs the area above the throat and the four limbs; it also controls the upward flow of energy in the body. Samana governs the navel area and the digestive processes. Uyana pervades the entire body; apana governs the area below the navel. Finally, prana governs the area between the throat and diaphragm, controlling respiration and speech functions. The skilled practitioner has to learn to distinguish and operate the five different forms of prana. According to Satyananda the conscious joining of prana and apana at the solar plexus is a very important practice, which serves to awaken this centre. The two different energies meet and generate great force.

Prana is universal to all living things. It is absorbed from living food, from the air itself and from unspoilt natural landscapes. This raises the single most important issue of our day: that of the pollution of our world, affecting the quality of the air we breathe and the food we eat.

Leslie Kenton, whose many books promote health, beauty and fitness suggests a way of life that centres upon living food, that is food that still carries prana. She has no doubts about the value of fresh raw vegetables and extracted juices as sources of vitamins and minerals. Bioenergetic foods—seeds, grains, nuts and pulses—along with fresh vegetables and fruit share one unique property: they each radiate life force.[1] Kirlian photography has given us some fascinating insights into this. When organic matter is fresh, it radiates a bright emanation. As it ages, these emanations fade in brightness and eventually disappear altogether. Foods that lack all traces of life force are ultimately destructive to the body. Living food enhances the whole being. A diet built around living food will contribute over a period of time to raise the vibrations of the subtle energies to a higher level.

This centre is given great importance in traditional Japanese teachings. It is called the hara, which literally means 'belly'. It is the centre point where all things both visible and invisible find their balance. The hara is traditionally located three fingers' width below the navel. When this chakra functions as the gravitational centre of being, emotions are both felt and expressed. When the powers of this centre are repressed, serious discrepancies between true feeling and action can arise. Anorexia is a disorder in which the gut feelings are denied and overlaid instead with a false self-image. When the hara is operative, unified expression through word, action and body language follow. In Japan a person is judged to be untrustworthy and insincere unless the voice comes from the hara.

Overtone singing is a fascinating and ancient way of reaching the energies of the hara. It can be liberating, even cathartic. Sit or stand keeping the back straight. Begin by breathing yogically. Put the tip of the tongue against the top of the mouth while inhaling. Exhale while your tongue curls slightly backwards. Let the air out without a sound. Your mouth should be positioned so that there is a small space between the tongue and the roof of your mouth. The tip of the tongue faces backwards. Let the sides of the tongue lightly touch the top teeth. Now you are ready to try for an overtone. Choose a comfortable tone and place it within the hara. When the sound is formed it can be varied by moving the position of the tongue inside the mouth and by altering the shape of the lips. When the overtone is sounded two notes are heard at the same time and there is a sensation of vibration in the head. Overtone chanting can provide a wonderful experience when performed in a group.

Awareness of this centre can also be developed through hara breathing. This involves bringing awareness to the centre while establishing a breathing rhythm. The hands are placed over the centre. At the same time the tongue is touched to the upper palate. This connects the governor and conceptual meridians and facilitates the flow of prana from the centre. While inhaling deeply to the count of five, a radiant light flowing in with the air is visualised. The breath is held for a count of five and the energy is felt accumulating at the centre. The air is exhaled for a count of five. An unbroken breathing rhythm is established. The exercise can be done while lying down for about twenty minutes. It brings a feeling of great bodily warmth and personal energy. In Tibet an advanced technique was evolved for generating body heat. Its name is Tummo. Prana is extracted from the vast natural reservoirs and stored in the human body in order to generate heat. The system employs elaborate meditation, complex visualisations, postures and breath control. The practitioner builds the form of a golden lotus at the navel and uses the bija mantra to invoke elemental fire. Fire is generated at the top of the head and drops down into the navel centre. In the mind's eye, the sushumna is increased in size until it encompasses the physical form. It becomes quite literally the channel for fire. After rigorous and long training, the candidate is tested by his teacher. Alexandra David-Neel, who travelled and studied in Tibet, described what she saw of Tummo in practice. 'The neophytes sit cross-legged and naked. Sheets are dipped in icy water. Each man wraps himself in one of them and must dry it on his body. As soon as the sheet has become dry, it is again dipped in the water as before. The operation goes on in that way until daybreak, then he who dried the largest number of sheets is acknowledged the winner of the competition.'[2]

In Tibetan 'repa' means 'the cotton clad one'. The great teacher Milarepa mastered Tummo under the guidance of his teacher Marpa. Milarepa was forced to overwinter in a freezing cave one year. He wrote a poem about his experience, ending with the lines:

The life and death struggle of the fighter could there be seen
And I, having won the victory, left a landmark for the hermits
Demonstrating the great virtue of Tummo.[3]

It is difficult to say whether such traditions have been lost with the destruction of the Tibetan way of life but there is adequate testimonial to the total mastery of heat and cold by masters of the past. This is but one expression of the powers of the manipura chakra, the solar plexus, the personal sun.

The solar plexus chakra is our place of empowerment in the world. It is the personal fuel store. If the fuel store is low, we lack the driving force to project ourselves into the world with impact. We become victims of fate and circumstance when we lose touch with will power which is a direct expression of inner being. The will is fundamental to well-being and personal fulfilment, translating our innermost nature into outer expression, enabling us to overcome difficult life circumstances. If an individual is weak-willed, the qualities of self-determination and self-direction are undeveloped. They are easily swayed from any given course by the influence of others. If someone is wilful, they exercise power with total disregard to others. It is through the expression of will that we create our own reality; our power in the world is an expression of our sense of will. The human will has been seen by many esoteric writers as a reflection of a divine attribute, the Primal Will, which brings creation into being. It is through the human will that change for good or evil comes into being in the world. We have free will; this gives us choice and teaches us the value of discrimination. It is through the conscious use of will that our lives are forged.

When the will is blocked we experience a sense of frustration which is often accompanied by a tightening of the whole solar plexus area. When we lose our sense of power, the stomach seems to turn to water. Our strength vanishes, our fire has been extinguished. Ideally there should be a free flow of energy between the personal will and the freedom to project in the world, but this is often blocked. It can be a temporary obstacle created by a personal dispute or it can be longer-lasting situation of repression. Accord between inner comprehension of personal will and outer freedom of expression allows the energy of the third chakra to flow evenly. When the will is blocked, either at source or externally, the chakra cannot release and energies begin to impact. The chakra acts like a dam holding back feelings, energies, needs and drives. There is inner turmoil, repressed anger and contained force. Eventually something snaps and there is an emotional scene, a crisis, even a breakdown. This chakra contains our raw emotions. When our emotions are freely expressed they pass easily from us into the appropriate situation and become integrated as part of our total being. When emotions, for whatever reason, are not expressed but turned inwards, they remain lodged in this chakra until catharsis takes place. Anger especially can remain trapped here for many years.

The stomach is very sensitive to sudden changes in our feelings. When we experience butterflies in the pit of our stomach we are experiencing fear or extreme nervousness. If we experience a sudden shock it can feel like a blow to the stomach and we feel physically sick. When we are upset we find it difficult to eat. These physical sensations are mirror images of the activity of the chakra itself.

This chakra represents an important step in the development of human consciousness. It carries no trace of our shared animal ancestry, unlike the base and sacral chakras. Some tantric teachings regard it as the starting point for higher human development for this very reason. Satyananda calls it the place of 'confirmed awakening', indicating that when this level is reached the Kundalini force will not sink back into the lower centres.

Traditionally the awakening of this chakra is said to bring the power to locate hidden treasure. This is an interesting correspondence with the actual name of this chakra, lustrous gem. It may also have a symbolic meaning indicating that spiritual reality itself is the hidden treasure. The awakening of this chakra is said to confer mastery over fire. This refers to the internal fires and to the generation of psychic heat through controlled use of natural energy. The ability to see the body from within is also said to develop as the functions of this chakra unfold. This is especially pertinent when we remember the training involved in Prana Vidya where visualisations focus on the internal anatomy as channels for the circulation of prana. The initiate functioning at this level is said to be able to send prana to the sahasrara chakra and to enjoy complete freedom from disease. This is only possible when a considerable degree of control has been achieved over prana.

When we look at the traditional images for this chakra, we find ten petals, coloured greenish-blue, the colour of a rain cloud. Each petal is inscribed with a consonant in bright blue. In the centre is a downward-pointing red triangle, the region of fire, with additional T-shaped projections at each edge to suggest movement. The bija mantra or seed sound for this chakra is ram, which is also coloured red. The ram, vehicle of Agni the god of fire, represents the fiery qualities of this chakra. One of the deities of this chakra is Rudra, an aspect of Visnu and Lakini. Rudra is the god of storms; he has both a vengeful and a benign aspect, indicating that power can be used both positively and negatively. Rudra is known as 'the red one'. He is often depicted as being ruddy in colour, but is also shown with a white face smeared with ashes.

Sakti Lakini is a form of Laksmi, the goddess of good fortune and beauty. She is usually portrayed either standing or seated upon a lotus. In this instance Lakini sits upon a red lotus. She is blue and has three faces with three eyes in each. The third eye symbolises the increased psychic sense that comes with the awakening of this chakra. She has four arms and holds a vajra—a thunderbolt symbolising power—and a sakti or fire weapon. She makes the signs for granting boons and dispelling fears. She has fierce projecting teeth and is fond of eating rice and dhal mixed with meat and blood. This again brings us back to the colour red.

The overwhelming visual symbolism of this chakra focuses the mind upon the element of fire and the colour red.

Physically this chakra governs the stomach and digestive system. The manipura chakra relates to the liver, gall bladder, stomach and spleen. Imbalances can give rise to eating or digestive disorders. Ulcers, which are frequently related to high levels of stress, are a classic disorder of this centre.

When the energies of this chakra are active and balanced, the individual enjoys well-being and has a clear sense of personal self-determination.

ORIENTATION EXERCISES

1. Explore the concept of personal power by considering how you use power in the world.
2. Meditate on the element of fire.

PRANAYAMA EXERCISES

1. JOINING THE STREAMS

1. Sit with a straight spine.
2. Inhale deeply. Imagine prana being absorbed through your throat and flowing down to your navel.
3. At the same time imagine apana flowing up from the muladhara to the navel. Assume mula banda (perineum lock) and visualise the two streams uniting at the navel.

You might also work on THE BREATH OF FIRE and HARA BREATHING.

ASANAS

1. BELLY PUSH

1. Sit with your legs outstretched, hands flat on the floor underneath your shoulders.

2. Lift your body by raising your buttocks.
3. Make a straight line with your body from the toes to the head.
4. Drop back to a seated position and repeat.

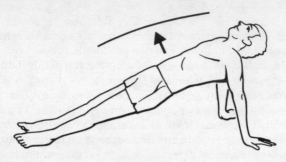

Belly Push

2. SPINAL FLEXES.

This exercise flexes the spine in both directions.
1. Sit on your heels with your hands on your knees and curve your back.
2. Inhale and arch your back. Push your chest up and out.
3. Exhale as you slump down. Repeat the cycle.

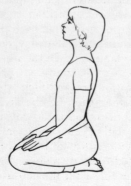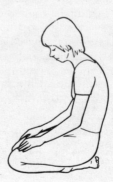

Spinal Flex

3. THE PINCERS (PASCHIMOTTANASANA)

1. Sit on the floor with your legs extended, arms on thighs.
2. Slowly bend your upper torso forwards, sliding your hands along the legs.

3. Bend forward as far as it comfortable; idealy the forehead should touch the knees.

VISUALISATION: GREETING THE SUN

Find yourself standing on a high outcrop of rock in a barren treeless landscape. It is still quite dark; dawn is about to break. Your vantage point enables you to look out across the land. Even in this light you are able to see a vast desert plain stretching in every direction. Here and there you see huge stony outcrops like fingers reaching up into the sky. At the distant edge of the horizon, the sun begins to rise. You watch as the great ball of fire shows itself. It seems red in colour as it comes into view. You raise your arms in greeting as this great being emerges from the darkness of night. Sunlight begins to flood the terrain, lighting up the seemingly endless vista. You feel a touch of warmth on your face as the sun's rays lengthen.

As the sun rises higher into the sky, changing in colour from red to a burning yellow, it seems to ignite the spark within your own fire centre. Your mind becomes filled with the image of a radiating sphere deep within your centre of being. It glows with brightness that spreads outward as you stand upon your high peak. It rises within you as a great fiery ball emerging from slumber. You begin to breathe deeply, drinking in the rays of the sun like a liquid gold. As you breathe in you are filled with a shower of brilliance. As you breathe out, you radiate this divine energy towards other living forms. As you stand in the ever-increasing brightness of a new day, become aware of the living quality of the whole landscape. In the freshness of the new dawn everything radiates life. As you continue with your deep breathing your inhalations seem to put you in touch with the very life force of the land, the stones, the sand and the air itself. As you breathe in you feel that you are drinking in the power that the land has to offer you, sharing in its daily cycle of renewal. This force fills your power centre, flooding you with vital life force. You feel wholly alive, empowered, exhilarated. Your own energy store is now full to overflowing. Take this power into your life and use it to be fulfilled.

DREAM IMAGES

This chakra produces a wide array of fiery images: setting a fire; preparing a ritual fire; watching a house on fire; even being on fire but paradoxically being unharmed, much like the burning bush. Images of sunrise or other solar images can be indicative of an awakening at this level.

BACH FLOWER REMEDIES

Aspen	2	Overcoming fears
Hornbeam	17	Being able to achieve personal goals
Impatiens	18	Patience
Larch	19	Self-awareness
Scleranthus	28	Balance within yourself
Star of Bethlehem	29	Ability to act from joy

MUSIC

This chakra is concerned with expressing emotions. When emotions are not released at the appropriate time the vibration quite literally becomes lodged in the chakra and the body. Music that has the power to express an emotion, whether it is grief or joy, can provide a much needed cathartic experience. You might like to listen to Sunrise by David Sun, The Enchanter by Tim Wheater and Aquamarine by Stairway.

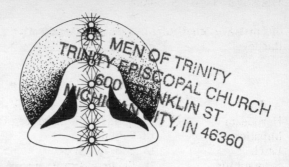

7 · THE GATEWAY OF THE WINDS

THE HEART CHAKRA: TABLE OF
CORRESPONDENCES

Location Rooted between the fourth and fifth thoracic vertebrae
Sanskrit name Anahata, meaning 'unstruck'
Element Air
Function Love
Inner state Compassion, love
Body parts Lungs, heart, arms, hands
Glands Thymus
Malfunction Asthma, blood pressure, heart disease, lung disease
Colour Green
Seed sound Lam
Sense Touch
Petals Twelve: kam, kham, gam, gham, ngam, cham, chham, jam, jham, nyam, tam, than
Animal symbols Antelope, birds, dove
Deities Isa, Kakini

He who meditates on this Heart lotus becomes like the Lord of Speech, and like Isvara he is able to protect and destroy the worlds.

Sat-Cakra-Nirupana, Verse 26

Rising up from the solar plexus we now encounter the heart chakra. Its name anahata means unstruck or unbeaten. It refers to a sound that

GOD: Isa   GODDESS: Kakini

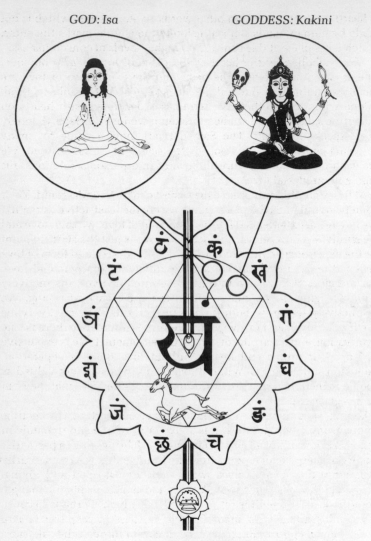

Anahata Chakra
From Kundalini Yoga far the West

is heard yet is not struck, in other words an eternal note which is not made by human hands. This allusion to the eternal marks the entry, which takes place at this centre, into higher levels of consciousness.

The symbolism of the heart as the place of love is also obvious. The associations between the heart and the experience of love are deeply engrained in our culture. It is almost impossible to think of one without the other. We send cards decorated with hearts on Valentine's day and we are heartbroken if we lose our love. A lonely heart speaks for itself. The Sacred Heart, now a name for many convents and schools, symbolises transcendent Christian love. We are each more familiar with the love of interpersonal relationships than with universal love.

At first sight this seems to be the easiest chakra to understand. Yet it often turns out to be the place where we are the least active in reality. We have each experienced falling in and out of love, we each love and are surely loved in return. Yet personal love is just the starting point for the experience of this chakra. The quality, degree and form of love assigned to the fourth chakra is quite different from personal love. For the most part we aim to bring love into our lives, instinctively acknowledging the goodness within the experience of loving. We instinctively recognise both its presence and its absence. Everyone needs to be loved and to give love in return. Without love there is true deprivation, and a warping of natural development. Love is expansive and open; it unites and heals. Without love there is separation, exclusion and coldness. Without love, individuals are not valued as people in their own right, they are simply exploited for what they can do in a given capacity.

Loving encompasses nurturing, caring, supporting, protecting, among many other qualities. It is active in principle and dynamic in action. Yet love is not an abstract intangible. It brings forth a particular quality of energy which pours from the heart centre. We momentarily experience this for ourselves when we are most open and loving. There can be a distinct physical sensation which seems to emanate from the heart. Sometimes it is almost like a pain. Perhaps because this level of intensity is uncomfortable, we tend to keep this chakra under mental control. Energy can be drawn in through the sahasrara chakra and then sent out through the heart to others. In this experience it is possible to become a channel for a particular quality of energy.

A few individuals live their whole lives in this way, radiating from the heart. This degree of loving is a rare thing. It is compassion, which is universal and unconditional love. It is a continuous flow of living energy through the heart chakra towards others. This energy itself has the power to heal and change. Mother Theresa is without doubt a living embodiment of this force; she is a channel for the love of Christ which flows through her. She wrote of this, 'Let Him empty and transform you and afterwards fill the chalice of your hearts to the brim, that you in your turn may give of your abundance.'[1]

The major processes for opening the heart are outlined in this deceptively simple statement. First the heart is emptied of selfish desires, preparing the way for transformation into a centre for selfless love. Finally the opened heart is like a chalice overflowing with living water, a constant stream of divine love.

The model of the selfless, all-loving, all-giving being is not confined to Christianity. Buddhism places great value on the development of universal compassion. It is here that we find the concept of the Bodhissatva, an enlightened being who forgoes Nirvana and instead remains out of compassion to bring liberation to others. This ideal has much in common with the ideal of becoming a Christed being. It represents the highest state of individual aspiration. The path towards Bodhissatvahood is clearly defined. It begins with an ordination ceremony and a code of conduct: 'I, (name) who have caused the thoughts of enlightenment to arise, accept the infinite world of living beings as my mother, father, sister, brother, son, daughter and any other blood relations, and having accepted them as far as in my power, strength and knowledge, I cause the roots of goodness to grow in them.'

By keeping the role model of the Bodhissatva constantly in the mind, by acting like a Bodhissatva according to a series of vows and undertakings, gradual transformation takes place. It is believed that His Holiness the Dalai Lama is an incarnation of Chenrezig, one of the compassionate Bodhissatvas.

There have always been those exceptional people who have been able to transcend the limitations that bind and blind others. It was Rumi, the greatest mystical poet of the Sufi tradition, who gave the world a glimpse of his vision of divine love through poetry. Like all mystics he saw the universe as a place of unbounded and overflowing love. Everything expressed this one principle.

Ramakrishna, who experienced the complete rising of Kundalini, found it difficult to convey the experiences of the higher centres even to his closest pupils. Simply talking about the mystical state immediately returned him to a state of ecstasy in which he was quite literally struck dumb. He did however one day describe the function of the heart chakra in the following way: 'In the scriptures mention is made of the seven centres of consciousness. When the mind is attached to worldliness, consciousness dwells in the lower three centres. There are no high ideals or pure thoughts. It remains in greed and lust. The fourth centre of consciousness is the region of the heart. Spiritual awakening comes when the mind rises to this centre. At this stage man has a spiritual vision of the divine light and is struck with wonder at its beauty and glory. His mind no longer runs after worldly pleasures.'[2]

Ramakrishna experienced the awakening of the higher centres as blissful states of ecstasy. He, like other mystics, felt he had personally encountered the universal field of love and the underlying unity of creation. Mystical experiences are difficult to explain, even to express, rather like having to explain a brief visit to a foreign country where few people have travelled before. Ordinary language cannot explain the experience, words cannot convey the essential meaning which far outstrips the limitations of words. The language of poetry, with its rich symbolism, is often the most appropriate means of expressing the ineffable. It often proves to be the natural language of the mystic.

When this centre awakens it is said to bring poetic genius and eloquence. The *Sat-Cakra Nirupana* tells us, 'Inspired speech flows like a stream of clear water.' Gopi Krishna, who experienced the awakening of Kundalini over a period of years, records the time when he became overtaken by a sudden and unexpected ability to write poetry. It followed close on the heels of a mystical experience which he described, thus: 'I had expanded in an indescribable manner into a titanic personality, conscious from within of an immediate and direct contact with an intensely conscious universe, a wonderful inexpressible immanence all around me . . . It was an amazing and staggering experience for which I can find no parallel and no simile, an experience beyond all and everything belonging to this world.'[3] Before coming completely out of this state poetry began to form in Gopi Krishna's mind. 'The lines occurred one after another, as if dropped into the three dimensional fields of my consciousness by another source of knowledge within me.'[4] He wrote in Kashmiri, English, Urdu, Punjabi, Persian, German, French, Italian, Sanskrit and Arabic, several of which were languages he had not studied.

The heart centre is not easy to fully awaken. Our love is so easily limited to family, friends, to those who love us in return. Many grow up in loveless and unloving homes and have no experience of being nurtured and valued. Even personalised love at its most giving and open-hearted is but a reflection of a universal and unlimited love.

By tradition this chakra holds the second knot called the vishnu granthi. To awaken this centre we have to dissolve our limited views of reality which restrict the flow of our love. The Katha Upanishad tells us that 'When all the knots of the heart are loosened, then even here in this human birth, the mortal becomes immortal. This is the whole teaching of the scriptures.'[5]

The heart centre is unique in having a subsidiary chakra, which is represented within a lotus of eight petals beneath the anahata chakra. This subsidiary chakra is called the Kalpavriksha or Kalpa tree and is known as the celestial wish-fulfilling tree. The place is described as an island of gems with a wonderful tree. There is a jewelled altar surmounted with an awning and decked with flags. It is here that the disciple may come and offer mental worship. It is said to function only when the anahata has been awakened first. This centre is said to grant personal wishes. Paradoxically if this centre has truly awakened, the heart's desire will be for the happiness and good of others.

The anahata centre controls the sense of touch. This is not surprising, for the heart meridians run along the length of the arms into the hands. It is through our hands that we offer love in the form of comfort, a loving caress or a healing touch. Prana is most easily radiated through the hands and with appropriate visualisation it can be directed from the heart centre itself. The individual develops an increasingly subtle sense of touch which enables the energy field of others to be directly sensed. At a workshop I attended we were each engaged in our own meditation on the heart chakra when I became aware of a strong sensation, almost a pain in my heart. Yet I knew that this was not my pain. Almost immediately I knew that it was emanating from the woman sitting across the room directly opposite me. Her distress and emptiness of heart was so painful that I consciously began to pour out waves of energy. My mind's eye seemed to see streams of light crossing the room. At the end of the session I went straight over to her and we shared our experiences. She instinctively knew that I had sent a healing light towards her, even though she had not opened her eyes during the meditation period and I had correctly intuited her deep distress.

The element relating to this chakra is air. Of all the elements this is the least tangible. We draw oxygen from the air quite unconsciously thousands of times every day. By contrast spiritual disciplines place great emphasis upon conscious breathing as part of mental training and expansion of consciousness. Most people breathe from the top of the lungs alone. Deep breathing, which uses as much lung capacity as possible, counteracts the tendency to live and breathe in a shallow manner. The deep breath has the effect of keeping us in touch with our feelings. Rebirthing, commences with conscious connected breathing as a way of reaching deep memories and feelings. The conscious breath is absolutely vital for a conscious life. There is a direct link between the control of the breath and the control of prana.

This chakra is described as having twelve vermilion petals. The yantra for this centre is a hexagonal star, the upward-pointing triangle of Shiva or consciousness meeting the downward-pointing triangle of Shakti or force. It is a smoky colour, like the faint stream of smoke that rises as incense is burned. At the centre of the star is a downward-pointing triangle containing a bana-linga in the form of crescent moon which symbolises the psychic blockage within this chakra. When this knot is dissolved it becomes possible to enter into the universal life.

The previous centres are closely bound up with personal and group karma. Opening the lower three chakras inevitably releases karmic forces. However the anahata chakra is not subordinate to karmic influences. The individual stands above and outside the bounds of karma. The path towards higher consciousness begins at this level, where karma no longer binds and universal life is experienced.

The intelligence of this level is symbolised by Isa, an aspect of Shiva and Kakini. Isa, shining white or brick red is called the lord of speech. He represents the whole world system in which the diversities of phenomenal realities of time and space are gradually revealed. He makes a gesture that grants boons and dispels fears. He carries nothing. Kakini, shining yellow, carries a noose and a skull. The noose reminds us not to become captured in the expectation of spiritual experience and the skull reminds us of the need to maintain a pure mind. She too makes a gesture that grants boons and dispels fears. The mantra for this chakra is Yam. The quality of this chakra is symbolised by a black antelope or gazelle, vehicle of Vayu, Vedic god of the winds. The gazelle, which leaps and bounds with consummate ease, symbolises the lightness of physical substance. It is a further reminder of the element of air.

The activation of this centre brings many different qualities. As this centre opens it brings an increasingly subtle sense of touch. The individual becomes highly sensitised to the energy fields of others and it becomes possible to detect areas where there is disturbance and disease simply through the refinement of touch. The ability to heal is a natural extension of the increased capacity for love. Prana is easily directed through the hands in a healing contact. Psychokinesis can also develop when the anahata awakens. The power to love impersonally and without discrimination remains the central quality of this chakra, however. It is from this expansion of love that all other qualities naturally flow.

Motoyama's invaluable personal record of his own awakening relates the opening of the heart chakra in the following way: 'One morning (while practising water asceticism by pouring cold water over himself in the cold early morning) the following occurred. I saw a great energy rising from my coccyx to my heart through the spine. My chest felt very hot and I saw my heart start to shine a brilliant gold. The icy water was warmed by this heat, steam rose from the surface of my body, but I did not feel cold . . . When I came to myself ten to twenty minutes later my mother told me that she had seen a golden shining light at the top of my head and at my heart. I think this experience is the point at which my anahata chakra awakened . . . Since then I have been able to do psychic healing. After the awakening of the anahata chakra then, I learned to control the abilities both to emit psi energy and to perform psychic healing. My psychological state also underwent some profound changes with this awakening; notably I developed an attitude of non-attachment to worldly things. I began to feel constant optimism about everything. My wishes were often spontaneously fulfilled.[6]

It is fascinating to note how this account confirms the traditional descriptions of the awakening of this chakra. Motoyama tells us, for example, of his increasing optimism. Satyananda reminds his students of the following: after the awakening and ascension of Kundalini to a given chakra, mental negativism will cause it to descend back into the base centre. Should it descend after having touched the anahata level, it will be increasingly difficult to reawaken. It is therefore essential that the student should not lose his or her optimism even for a moment in order to keep Kundalini shakti at the anahata level. This reminds us that we cannot study the chakras individually without also considering their complex relationship to Kundalini herself. As the chakras become more active, so Kundalini awakens and further opens the receiving chakras in an endless cycle of action and reaction.

When this chakra is open and balanced there is a genuine ability to give and to receive. Compassion develops and becomes a natural expression of feeling.

ORIENTATION EXERCISES

1. Explore your own experiences of giving and receiving love.
2. Meditate on the element of air.

ASANAS

1. FLAPPING WINGS

1. Stand with your arms outstretched.
2. Stretch your arms backwards without bending the elbows so that you feel a pressure in your shoulder blades.

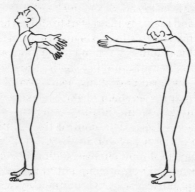

Flapping Wings

3. Keep bending your hands backward.
4. Inhale and raise your chest up and outwards. Exhale: keeping the arms outstretched bring your palms together in front of you, curving the spine slightly forward.
5. Take your hands back on the inhalation.
6. Bring them forward on the exhalation.

This wonderfully dynamic exercise is helpful for releasing constrictions in the chest area. It stimulates the points normally used to treat cardiovascular problems. It also counteracts rounded shoulders and slumped postures, which are so often produced by sedentary work.

2. CROSSING THE HEART

1. Sit cross-legged if possible.
2. Place your right hand in the left armpit and your left hand in the right armpit.
3. Close your eyes and feel your heart beating.
4. Attempt to locate the heart space and meditate upon it. The vision of the blue lake and blue lotus may appear during this pose.

3. OPENING THE HEART

1. Stand straight, with the feet shoulder-width apart.
2. Breathe deeply and raise the arms above the head.
3. Bend backward, letting the head drop back. If you find this difficult, stand near a wall for support. Do not hold this pose for more than a few seconds at first. This is a surprisingly dynamic exercise which instantly reveals areas of restriction.

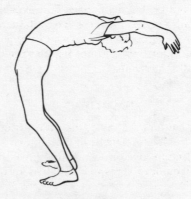

Opening the Heart

VISUALISATION: THE ROSE OF THE HEART

Allow the mind to become quiet. Focus your awareness upon the area of the physical heart and its cavity. Although the physical heart occupies only a small space, the true heart is without limitations. Try to feel the beating of your own heart. Begin to think of the people that you are able to love. Allow their faces to rise up singly so that you are able to acknowledge each one individually. As you do this you may feel a sensation even a tightness around the heart. Look into the heart space and see the bud of a rose slowly unfolding. Watch the slow movement of the petals as the bloom grows within you. Continue to think about the people whom you love. Now think of those who love you. Watch the rose increasing in size. See the softness of the petals and beauty of its fresh bloom. Allow the rose to complete its growing until it seems to fill your heart. Now radiate the love that you have accumulated. Let it stream out from the heart in a shaft of bright light. Let your love pour forth in a steady stream to those whose hearts are empty.

FINDING THE HEART SPACE

Sit in a comfortable position for meditation. Close the eyes and concentrate on the throat. Breathe in with a deep full breath. Feel the breath filling the chest cavity. Allow the outgoing breath to pass without attention. Repeat this until you are fully focused on the breath. Next direct your attention to the space just above the diaphragm. Become aware of this space being filled. Gradually you will develop an awareness of this heart space. When you feel that you have discovered it, the heart space will expand and contract in time with the breath. If consciousness is maintained, the student will spontaneously see a vision of a blue lake and a blue lotus. This vision will appear at the right time. Do not use the power of the creative imagination to build the scene.

DREAM IMAGES

The heart chakra can appear in dreams in a variety of ways. These dreams typically involve scenarios in which love is a central theme: being in love, falling in love or even losing love. Such dreams often evoke a keenly-felt emotional response such as joy or deep sadness.

BACH FLOWER REMEDIES

Centuary	4	Service
Chicory	8	Overcoming distance
Heather	14	Unconditional love
Holly	15	Free-flowing love energy
Honeysuckle	16	Living in the here and now
Red chestnut	25	The ability to express true love
Rock rose	26	Overcoming ego limitations

MUSIC

This centre is concerned with making contact with the universalised power of love. Everyone is familiar with certain pieces of music which have the power to melt the heart. The natural sounds of whales and dolphins can take us beyond ourselves. Pachelbel's *Canon* which is often used for circle dancing is a wonderfully soothing and healing piece of music. You might also like to listen to these pieces with the heart, not the mind: *Great Piece* by Robert Martin, *Quiet Water* by Fitgerald and Flanagan, *The Response* by John Richardson, *Edge of Dreams* by Phil Thornton and *Deep Enchantment* by David Sun.

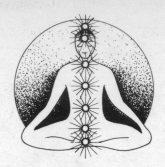

8 · THE GATEWAY OF TIME AND SPACE

Location The throat
Sanskrit name Vishuddi, meaning 'to purify'
Element Akasa
Function Creativity, communication
Inner state Intuition, synthesis
Body parts Neck, shoulders
Glands Thyroid and parathyroid
Malfunction Sore throat, swollen glands, colds, thyroid problems
Colour Bright blue
Seed sound Ham
Sense Hearing
Petals Sixteen: A, Ā, I, Ī, U, Ū, Ṛ, Ṛ, L, Ḷ, E, ai, O, au, am, ah
Animals Elephant
Deities Sadasiva; Sakini, an aspect of Gauri

This region is the gateway of great Liberation for him who desires the wealth of Yoga and whose senses are pure and controlled.

Sat-Cakra-Nirupana, verse 30

GOD: Sadasiva   GODDESS: Gauri (Eternal)

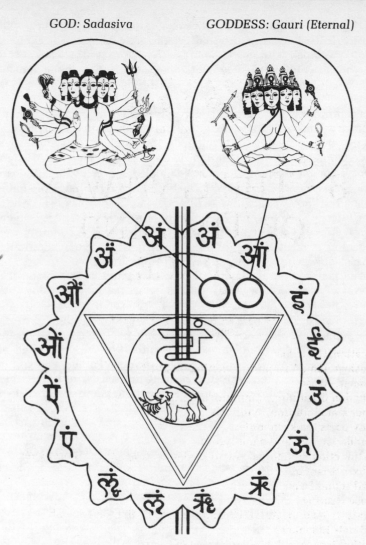

Visuddi Chakra
From Kundalini Yoga for the West

We have now reached the throat chakra, vishuddi. Its name means 'to purify'. This chakra is traditionally depicted with sixteen bright blue petals inscribed with vowel sounds. The yantra for this chakra is a downward-pointing triangle containing a circle, the akasamandala. The mantra for this chakra is Ham and the element for this centre is akasa.

The throat chakra represents our power to communicate verbally. The development of speech is unique to humanity, even though many other species have developed subtle and sophisticated ways of communication. Speech and the wide range of human vocalisation permit communication of a complex and unique kind. The human voice can convey emotion, information and a huge range of subtle meanings. We can sing, shout, whisper or laugh; we can cry or scream. The human voice can conceal the truth or reveal the truth. It is often possible to detect a lie in the voice; there is a lack of certainty and a quality of falsity. Great orators can inspire the group mind and demagogues can lead the group mind into madness.

The poet, writer and storyteller all instinctively understand the power of the word, whether spoken or written, and employ this power to evoke a personal response. Those working in mass media also understand the persuasive powers of communication and use the vehicle of the word to shape group consciousness. We are surrounded, indeed submerged, by words. We live in an age of mass communication and mass communicators. Paradoxically, this sea of sound has the effect of deadening our senses, dulling rather than sharpening our powers of discrimination, blunting rather than sharpening our critical faculties. Spiritual traditions have on the other hand kept alive the value of the word by preserving a place for silence through non-verbal contemplative practices. It remains only too easy to speak without thinking, to waste words and to utter empty phrases. Discovering the power of effective genuine communication is one of the tasks presented by this chakra.

Sound is vibration, an invisible energy. Both Christianity and Hinduism contain statements that affirm the creative, indeed the cosmic, power of sound. The gospel of St John tells us, 'In the beginning was the word and the word was with God and the word was God.' In the Vedas we find, 'In the beginning was Brahman with whom was the word and the word is Brahman.'

C. S. Lewis used this idea with good effect in his children's book, *The Magician's Nephew* when Aslan the lion sings creation into being. Tolkien, a contemporary of Lewis, also elaborated this idea in the *Silmarillion*. In the opening chapter we meet the Ainur, the Holy

Ones, offspring of the thoughts of Iluvatar. Each sings, fashioning the theme of Iluvatar to create a great music. Finally Iluvatar shows them what they have created. 'And as they looked and wondered this world began to unfold its history and it seemed to them that it lived and grew.'[1]

Tolkien's treatment is truly magical. In his evocative opening divine thought is translated into sound embodied in the Ainur, who in their turn create dense matter. We observe a descent of power from the spiritual to the physical, from the abstract to the concrete. Tolkien expresses a universal metaphysical belief in a hierarchical universe of descending vibrational states. The physical plane is the end result of the process of manifestation. It becomes separated from the source as well as other higher levels of vibration by the very nature of the creation process.

The compelling qualities of sound also exercised the minds of our predecessors who saw a reflection of the sacred in the elusive yet powerful nature of the word. Some three thousand years ago a philosophy and practice of sound was already well established in the Vedas and Tantras of eastern tradition. Such knowledge was part of a closely-guarded oral system of transmission. This teaching has survived probably in a truncated form as mantras.

There are many mantras, either single words or short phrases. These are used much like meditations. The individual becomes totally absorbed in the mantra at all levels of being. The mantra is sounded at the physical level but its effect is not confined to the mere physical sound of the word. It affects the whole being. The most well-known mantras are the Hindu 'Om' and the Buddhist 'Om mane padme hum'. Each of the chakras has its own bija mantra or seed sound. This sound is said to have the power to awaken the forces of the chakra. The individual mantra is vibrated and mentally placed within the appropriate chakra. The bija mantras, in ascending order starting at the base chakra are: lam, vam, ram, yam, ham and om. There is no bija mantra for the crown chakra.

John Diamond has investigated the relationship between sounds and meridian strength through muscle testing. He has discovered that certain sounds correspond to particular meridians, and that a meridian can be temporarily strengthened just after a sound has been vibrated.[2]

The function of hearing is assigned to this chakra, and refers to a subtle quality of inner hearing which is quite different from our ordinary day-to-day physical hearing. Motoyama wrote about his own experience in the following way. 'It is said that when the vishuddi awakens, the hearing becomes sharp; in fact I have had a lot of difficulty hearing due to tympanitus of both ears which started when I was a child; in addition the eardrum and the small bones in my left ear were surgically removed when I was young. However, since the vishuddi awakened I have been able to hear much more clearly, not with my physical ear, but with that of the mind.'[3]

By tradition the opening of this chakra brings increased telepathic rapport. Telepathy can be thought of as hearing inwardly, which is something that we all do from time to time. Usually this is no more than a fleeting, often unconscious experience. It is rarely under conscious control. The activation of this chakra, however, brings telepathy into consciousness. This level of inner hearing or mental rapport is quite different from the telepathy represented on the svadisthana level, which is essentially astral and symbolic in form, often being received as images and impressions. Telepathy at the mental level is direct, bypassing symbolic intermediaries. Mind meets mind. The fusing of thoughts can be instantaneous as it was with Alice Bailey, amanuensis for the Tibetan. Their joint undertaking – his thoughts received through her mind and meticulously recorded – produced a huge collection of esoteric literature. She described the process as a form of internally-heard dictation. From the outset she knew that she was in contact with a mind outside her own.

Channelling, telepathic communication with highly-evolved beings is now something of a phenomenon in the United States. Despite its rapid appearance over the last few years, there is nothing new in channelling except the name. Mediums, mediators and awakened individuals through the centuries have been able to make contact with discarnate beings. Such activity invariably arouses either hostility or sheer disbelief and in the past has been confined to esoteric or spiritualist groups. The current North American experience is quite different. It is open and highly public. Practitioners unhesitatingly claim to be in contact with a wide range of ancient, evolved and sometimes extra-terrestrial beings whose messages uniformly express concern and alarm at the benighted state of our planet.

It is only too easy to dismiss this phenomenon as a form of psychic mass hysteria in response to the genuine threat that is now posed to planetary life. However, channelling is but one expression in a long history of inner plane contact. It is impossible to say how much is genuine. The Tibetan estimated that of the material purported to come from the Masters only about two percent genuinely comes directly from that source. He further reminds the student of the need to discriminate between the vibration of his own soul, the vibration of the group with which he is associated and the vibration of the Master. Vibration is of course a key word in this case. We are reminded yet again of sound as the vehicle for vibration and also of the need to refine and develop the quality of inner hearing as the means of discrimination.

As the higher chakras open within the group as a whole we can expect more not less communication from the non-physical levels. Many people will find such concepts plainly unbelievable if not somewhat ridiculous. However such mediation is perfectly in accord with our knowledge of the chakras. The current North American experience may appear faintly ridiculous at times but in theory such communication is perfectly possible.

There is a link between the development of inner hearing and the process of creativity. Creative artists often perceive themselves as receivers tuned in to a particular wavelength which is not of their making. Some writers experience a kind of inner dictation; others have inspirational dreams. Musicians invariably hear music inwardly. The creative process can be like a powerful overshadowing or possession. So often the creative artist admits to feeling like an instrument of a greater power which in every respect appears to be external.

Esoteric teachings tell us that when the throat chakra is inactive, our creativity will likewise be subdued. We will be unable to hear inwardly, or outwardly to give form to originality. In other words we are inoperative as creative channels.

When we look at the Tree of Life we find that Daath corresponds to the throat chakra. Daath is particularly interesting. For a long time it was not accorded the full status of a sephirah, as though Daath consciousness itself was not consolidated. On the Tree of Life Daath is situated above the abyss, a departure point to inner space. Its title is Knowledge. Daath perfectly symbolises the search for knowledge through the exploration of both inner and outer space. Daath can be thought of as a portal in space, or perhaps in the contemporary image of a black hole. It can even be seen as a doorway into the reverse, negative side of the Tree. This level of consciousness can be frightening, for the familiar and the comforting cannot be found. It is a step into the abyss of unknowing. The circle within the yantra for this chakra is called the akasamandala, the Gateway of Liberation; it is the place of the void. Motoyama experienced the fear associated with stepping out into the unknown: 'I found myself facing an abyss of absolute void,

I experienced such a terrible fear that I wanted to stop Yoga. I often felt that my attachment to this world was coming to an end; that I was leaving this world through the experience.'[4] Motoyama overcame his fear by total surrender and went on to experience the positive aspects of his awakening.

Activation of the throat chakra is said to bring complete indestructibility. It is said to bestow a full knowledge of the Vedas and gives understanding of the past, present and future. It gives the powers to endure without food or drink and awakens the power of telepathy.

These powers are by no means as absurd as they might appear to be at first sight. The power of indestructibility does not refer to physical indestructibility but to an initiatory experience of a very high order. Such an experience confers the certain and absolute knowledge that consciousness itself cannot be destroyed or harmed under any circumstances.

Motoyama had the experience of standing outside time, 'I was able to see the past, the present and the future in the same dimension by surpassing the distinction between them. When I now gave spiritual consultation to members of the Shrine I could see their previous lives, their present situation and their future conditions as a continuous stream.'[5]

The vishuddi chakra functions in conjunction with two other minor centres, the lalana at the base of the nasal orifice and the bindu vishargha at the top of the brain towards the back of the head. Hindu monks are usually shaven except for a small tuft of hair which marks this spot. Its name means 'the falling of drops'. The sahasrara chakra secretes drops described as nectar which collect within the bindu. These then pass on to the lalana at the base of the nasal orifice. If the vishuddi has been awakened the drops undergo purification and then have the power to rejuvenate the body. As the divine nectar is purified, extraordinary metabolic control becomes a possibility. Yogis have in the past been buried for as long as forty days to test themselves in a state of suspended animation. In preparation for this trial, the tendon beneath the tongue is gradually severed so that the tongue is curled back in the epiglottis to seal the respiratory passage. This directly stimulates the lalana to secrete more nectar which falls to the vishuddi where it is distributed throughout the body.

In a Tokyo institute this hypothesis was tested in a series of experiments which confirmed the relationship between the awakened vishuddi, the lalana and bindu centres in matters of metabolic control.[6]

The intelligence of this level is symbolised by Sadasiva in an androgynous aspect. Half of his body is as white as snow, the other half is golden. His name means ever-beneficent. He has five faces with three eyes in each face and ten arms. He wears a garland of snakes and is clothed in a tiger's skin. He carries nine items: a noose (pasa), a goad (ankusa), the great snake (nagendra), a trident (sula), a flame (dahana), a bell (ghanta), a diamond sceptre (vajra), a sword (khadga) and a battle axe (tanka). He makes the abhayamudra gesture, which dispels fear. The noose again reminds us of the dangers of being caught in spiritual pride, the goad shows us that further effort is still required. The snake king symbolises wisdom, the trident symbolises the unity of the physical, etheric and causal bodies. The flame represents the fires of Kundalini. The bell symbolises the quality of inner hearing. The diamond sceptre symbolises indestructibility. The sword symbolises the necessary quality of discrimination and the battle axe serves to cut away the old aspects of self.

Sakti Sakini is clothed in yellow. She is the form of light itself. She is an aspect of Gauri, Mother of the universe and the other half to Lord Shiva's body. The note of androgeny that we find introduced here is interesting. The god names applied to Daath are Jehovah and Elohim. Both names are translated as God. Elohim is the title of God used in Genesis. It is feminine noun with a masculine plural termination affixed. A closer translation of Elohim might be 'gods and goddesses' or 'god' which is both feminine and masculine. Both the eastern and western systems indicate that at this level polarities are but manifestations of the one force.

Sakini carries a bow and arrow, a noose and a goad. She has five faces and four hands. The animal associated with this chakra is the moon-white elephant Airavata, vehicle of the god Indra. We saw this animal first at the base chakra wearing a black collar to indicate servitude. Now the collar has been removed and servitude has been transformed into service.

When this chakra is open and balanced the powers of communication and creativity come to life, adding a new dimension to our comprehension of experience.

ORIENTATION EXERCISES

1. Explore your own powers of communication by reflecting on what you say and how you say it.
2. Meditate on the element of Akasa.

ASANAS

1. SIDE TO SIDE

1. Lie comfortably on your back; inhale deeply.
2. Exhale and slowly turn your head to the left.
3. Inhale as your head returns to the centre.
4. Exhale as you turn your head to the right.
5. Continue this exercise for one minute, gently stretching your neck from side to side.

This simple exercise opens up the neck and stimulates the thyroid gland.

2. BRIDGE

1. Lie comfortably on your back with your legs bent and the bottoms of your feet flat on the floor; keep your hands by your sides.
2. Inhale bringing your arms up over your head to rest on the floor behind you.
3. Lift your pelvis upwards.
4. Exhale and lower your body down to the starting position.
5. Exercise for one minute.

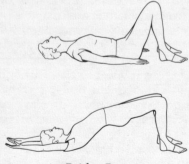

Bridge Pose

3. SHOULDER STAND

1. Lie down on your back; inhale and bend your knees towards your chest.
2. Exhale and swing your legs upwards so that your hips lift up from the floor.

3. Use your hands to support your lower back.
4. Straighten your legs and your back as much as possible.
5. Begin long, deep breathing.

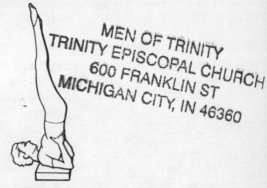

Shoulder stand

This asana causes subtle changes in the prana flow in the body and it facilitates the flow from manipura to vishuddi. This is also an important posture for transferring sexual energies from the lower to the higher dimensions. This asana should not be performed during menstruation. It should be performed with a firm support, either a foam Yoga block or a folded blanket placed beneath the shoulders, so that the neck and throat are slightly lower than the shoulders before the posture starts. This prevents the throat becoming constricted during the posture.

AWAKENING THE BINDU-VISHARGA

1. Sit in a meditational pose with the eyes closed.
2. Be aware of the natural breathing for some two minutes.
3. Use the mantra 'so ham'. Repeat 'so' on the inbreath and 'ham' on the outbreath. Place the sound in the throat.
4. Maintain awareness of the breath and the mantra together in a continuous rhythm.
5. Place the mantra in a straight line between the throat and a point at the top of the head towards the back.
6. On the inhalation imagine a thread of white light extending from the vishuddi to the bindu.

As these centres awaken, psychic sound, which is inaudible to physical hearing, can be heard around the bindu. This will indicate its location more precisely.

VISUALISATION: THE WOMB OF SPACE

Allow your surroundings to dissolve. Imagine that you stand before a great white wall. Step closer and place your hands upon it. You will find that it is not dense and solid but light as if made from a gossamer fabric stretched taught. Place your hands gently against the soft surface and feel it billowing against your hands. Take hold of the substance with both hands. Allow the wish to pass through the veil to rise within you.

As the thought is created so the veil opens between your hands creating a doorway shaped like a vesica piscis. You look beyond the veil and see the darkness and the wonder of deep space lit by points of white light. You make a choice to step back and close the veil or to step out into the unknown.

If you decide to return, simply step back and close the veil. If you wish to carry on step out with trust. You float in the silence of space. You are supported by space itself. The sensation is disconcerting, but if you surrender to your weightlessness you can begin to enjoy the new experience. You float effortlessly observing what you can in this strange silent world. Bright stars pepper the sky in every direction; some seem so close that you feel you might be able to touch them.

As you float you suddenly and unexpectedly become aware of a sound. It startles you momentarily. It is a note that seems to come from everywhere at once. Now you lie back and listen, trying to hear the sound more clearly. The note seems to swell in volume and to become more complex in some way. You are surrounded by the sound, which continues to reverberate. Now a new sound emerges. It is the sound of your name. You hear your name in a new way yet you cannot fail to recognise the vibration which is your name. You may answer if you wish, not with your voice but with your mind. The sound repeats over and over again like a mantra deep in space.

You seem able to sense the vibrations which your name creates. Your body begins to sway gently, rocked by unseen patterns of sound. You no longer float without direction. The power of sound carries you along on a wave which rises and falls with the patterns of your name. Your body sways on this sea of sound, gently propelled along by the vibrating notes themselves. Your body itself begins to vibrate. Your whole being takes up the resonance in harmony with the sounds that support you. As the resonance deepens you feel as if the very sound sloughs away the outworn and superfluous aspects of your existence which cling to you like a second skin. The sound continues its cleansing process, raising your vibrations to the pure sound of your true name. Now you seem to be moving along with ease propelled by waves of sound.

Ahead of you see the white gossamer veil with the open portal. Your journey nears its end. You have a last opportunity to express something, to speak with your inner voice. You reach the portal, carried gently all the way. You simply step through the opening and touch terra firma again. It feels good to return but it also feels good to have journeyed.

DREAM IMAGES

The images which relate to this chakra most often involve visits to highly unusual, foreign or strange places: mountain tops, hidden lands, undiscovered territories or quite alien landscapes. In such dreams contact is often made with a foreign race that appears to be superior in wisdom and understanding. Teaching is often offered either formally or informally. In the dream the content of this teaching carries great weight, yet paradoxically it seems difficult to recall it upon waking.

BACH FLOWER REMEDIES.

Agrimony	1	Fusing thinking and feeling
Mustard	21	Trusting your self even in the face of adversity
Wild oat	3	Communicating from your deepest levels
Willow	38	Making space for creativity

MUSIC

This centre expresses both the creativity of the individual and the spaciousness of the group. Immerse yourself in the sound of massed voices whether choirs or sacred chant. Lose yourself in the whole and paradoxically find your own note.

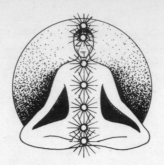

9 · THE GATEWAY OF LIBERATION

Location The brow, just above the bridge of the nose
Sanskrit name Ajna, meaning 'to know', 'to perceive' or 'to command'.
Element None applicable
Function Direct perception
Inner state Self-mastery
Body parts Eyes, two hemispheres of the brain
Gland Pituitary
Malfunction Headaches, nightmares, defects of vision
Colour Indigo
Seed sound Om
Sense None applicable
Petals Two
Animals None applicable
Deities Paramasiva (Shiva in the highest form) and Sakti Hakini

Within this lotus dwells the subtle mind.

Sat-Cakra-Nirupana, verse 33

We now rise up to the centre commonly associated with the third eye, the ajna chakra. This chakra has only two petals. These are inscribed with the mantras ham and ksham in white. These are the bija mantras of Shiva and Shakti respectively. The chakra is symbolised by a circle

GOD/GODDESS: Sakti Hakini

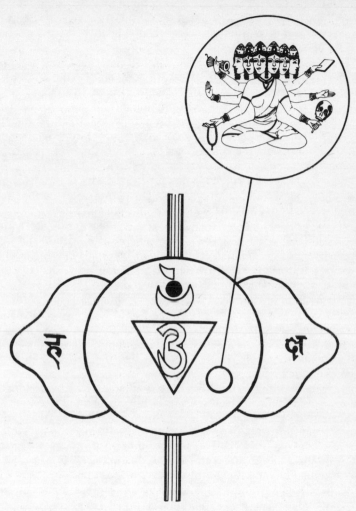

Ajna Chakra
From Kundalini Yoga for the West

containing the yantra for this chakra, a downward-pointing triangle which is golden in colour. The mantra for this chakra is om. Behind the mantra we see a linga named itara, white with streaks of lightning indicating power and energy. The deities of this chakra are Sakti Hakini and Shiva.

The name ajna is derived from Sanskrit roots meaning 'to know' and 'to follow'; it therefore means 'to command'. The ajna chakra may be thought of as the command centre of the whole being. This notion is especially significant for all would-be students in the mysteries. The spiritually-realised individual rules from 'the throne between the eyebrows' as Alice Bailey reminds us. In other words, life is under the control of a high level of consciousness and awareness.

The ajna chakra is located at the junction of the ida, pingala and sushumna meridians, at the brow. The confluence of the three energies brings extraordinary gifts once awakened. Sushumna alone rises upwards into the crown. Ida and pingala terminate at this junction. This is the underlying truth behind the idea of the third eye with which so many people are familiar. This centre certainly acts as a third eye when awakened. Its name 'to know' refers to aspects of telepathy and other means of direct knowing which bypass the ordinary senses. At this level immediate perception is a possibility. The barriers which circumscribe the self have long since been transcended. Just as a sighted person in a crowd of blind people would naturally have the advantage that sight brings, the awakened ajna chakra is the eye of the soul bringing all-round vision.

This chakra holds the last of the psychic knots, the knot of Shiva, the Rudra Granthi. This must be dissolved before the Kundalini serpent can rise fully and awaken the crown chakra. These knots can be understood as forces which bind and hold together the various levels of being. They have a most important function. When the appropriate levels of consciousness have been inwardly established the psychic knots no longer inhibit expansion. These might also be thought of as safety doors which are closed for protection. They will naturally open when the individual has gained a deep understanding of the forces concealed beyond the door. The key cannot be given by anyone, it has to be personally constructed. To dissolve this knot is to attain a state of unity, to overcome duality, to realise fully that there is no separation between self and everything else.

We see this represented in the traditional symbols for the ajna chakra which is depicted by two petals on either side of a circle.

The circle is Shunya, the void, and it is symbolised by white light. The void is beyond time and space; it is not empty but a state of pure existence; the void is the pure ground of being, the source and the point of return for manifestation.

The deity for this chakra is especially interesting. Sakti Hakini is both male and female: on the right side the figure is male, on the left the figure is female. This androgynous image is similar to the figure on the tarot trump XXI, the World, where we see a figure which is both male and female dancing within the realms of manifestation. Each aspect has its own mantra: ham is the mantra for the male aspect while sa is the mantra for the female aspect. Taken together, the mantra means 'I am that I am.' The God name for Kether, which more accurately relates to the crown chakra, is Eheieh which is also translated as 'I am that I am.'

The circle symbolising the void has two petals, one at each side. These can be thought of as the primal duality which proceeds from the unified state. This duality is present at all levels and even manifests within the physical form. The brain itself has two hemispheres, each with different and specialised functions. This basic polarity continues: the two eyes are connected to the different hemispheres of the brain, the outer body itself is symmetrical. This polarity also functions at very subtle levels. The overall energy field of the body can be thought of as an ovoid which extends outward from the body in all directions. However, the body, much like a bar magnet, produces sub-fields which flow in opposite directions. The chakras themselves form the mid line of the energy field where the two forces meet. Each chakra produces an energy field which reflects the activity within the centre itself. When the body is healthy, the energy field conforms to this basic pattern. Disease produces dead areas where the energy does not flow at all.

The image of the circle and the two petals is reminiscent of the winged solar disc of the Egyptians, a circle with wings on either side. This is an image of flight, freedom and liberation. It is also a symbol of a high cosmic initiation with which the Egyptians were familiar. The awakening of the ajna chakra can be viewed as an initiation, another step upon the journey of self awareness. The initiation of the ajana chakra brings the aspirant into contact with a 'supreme, eternal, birthless' state. When Motoyama awakened this chakra he found himself filled with ecstasy. He then became aware of a widened and deepened consciousness. In this state past, present and future were simultaneously known to him.

It is also said that this state of consciousness brings contact with the inner teacher, the source of wisdom within. The whole question of inner teachers is a particularly interesting one. Taking either the chakras or the sephiroth of the Tree of Life as a working guide, there can be no doubt that the small self of the personality makes contact with sources outside the limited self. These fall into two major groups, namely inner and outer teachers. The experience of the Holy Guardian Angel is essentially an experience of the higher self. This begins at Malkuth with the vision of the Holy Guardian Angel. This sephirah corresponds to the base chakra. At Tiphareth, which corresponds to the heart chakra, the initiate experiences the knowledge and conversation of the Holy Guardian Angel. The contact is externalised simply because consciousness at both Malkuth and Tiphareth remains within a dualistic paradigm. The ajna chakra corresponds to Binah, which is Wisdom, and Hokmah, which is Understanding. These two sephiroth individually represent the primary mother and father energies at a supernal level. We see this duality reflected in the two hemispheres of the brain which are yin and yang to one another. The awakening of the ajna chakra brings a contact with a source of wisdom which is experienced internally, as part of a oneness. The small self is absorbed into universalised wisdom; there is no sense of separation.

Outer teachers are also encountered as consciousness expands. These represent other minds developing upon their own path. Contact can be made with such minds as the inner mental faculties sharpen and develop. These minds too will become part of the oneness experienced through the ajna chakra. At lower levels of consciousness such minds also appear externally and will identify themselves as being individualised.

When we work with the chakras we come face to face with fundamental questions such as, What is the nature of self? What is the nature of reality? Experience is the only touchstone.

This is the first of the chakras to have its physical counterpart in the brain rather than in the body. The mind does not suffer from physical restrictions, but thoughts have wings. We can recreate the past from memory; we can plan for the future in our imagination; we can train the mind through meditation; we can experience a world of fantasy in our dreams.

As consciousness expands we discover new ways of using the mind. The activation of this chakra increases the powers of visualisation, which can be thought of as the power to see with the mind's eye. We each have a natural facility for creating images; the mind spontaneously produces images as part of the dreaming process. Children often have a vivid imagination which inevitably dulls with maturation and education. We were each once children with vivid imaginations, but we have invariably lost the quality to react to the world in a whole way, substituting instead the representational code of words rather than pictures. The value of visualisation seems to lie in its ability to involve the whole person in any given response. The picture-making facility has the power to evoke not merely the image itself but also a constellation of emotions and feelings. The image-producing abilities are centred in the right hemisphere of the brain, which is also responsible for emotional responses and symbolic representations of the world. It seems to be this fact which makes visualisation such a powerful tool in so many respects. Visualisation is a key component in certain forms of meditation. It is a significant factor in self-healing and in psychic unfoldment.

You can easily try out the power of visualisation for yourself in a small way. Start by naming something out loud for yourself. It could be anything simple such as a rose, a car or a tree. When you have named your chosen item, study your own response. What response did this word evoke from you? Now close your eyes and see a picture of the same item with the mind's eye. Create the image as clearly as you can and evaluate the image in the same way. What response did the image evoke from you? Now compare the effect of the spoken word with that of the created image. You will surely notice a qualitative difference in your own response. When visualisation is allied to real-life issues it has the power to evoke a deep-seated response which represents the total will of the individual. When visualisation is allied to everyday thinking it seems to open the door to new levels of perception and awareness. If you visualise an image of your friend before phoning, the way the image forms in your mind might prove to be informative. If you have a genuine need for something in your life, spend time creating the relevant image in your mind on a regular basis. When your mind is familiar with thinking visually, it seems to create an internal blank screen, ever ready for the spontaneous projection of images. When images arise in this way one part of the mind seems to produce a picture which it then hands over to another part of the mind for interpretation.

The whole process of visualisation from the neurophysiological roots to the sublime spiritual heights is now of such interest that scientists are keen to explore it further, doctors are willing to use it and psychiatrists take it seriously as a valuable tool in the regaining the wholeness of the psyche. Spiritual disciplines have always used visualisation as a key process in mental training and the expansion of consciousness. As speech is to the throat chakra, so visualisation is to the brow chakra.

The mind has the power to transcend limitations. We sometimes see this clearly demonstrated. Christy Brown, crippled from birth became an outstanding writer. He could not speak and could only control his left big toe. Yet his mind was alive and totally aware. The brilliant scientist Stephen Hawking suffers from a debilitating physical disease but his mind is incisive and has enabled him to revolutionise ideas about black holes. Here is a man who is confined to a wheelchair, yet he is able to contemplate the mysteries of deep space. His situation is a powerful symbol of the liberating power of the ajna chakra.

The ajna chakra brings freedom at many levels. Its liberation lies in the fact that it represents a state of consciousness in which there are no divisions and no limitations. It is outside and beyond all constraints. The state of consciousness represented by the ajna chakra is also beyond all personal karmic influences. The individual who has awakened the forces of the ajna chakra is able to use the energies to help the karmic situation of others. This is a most extraordinary concept which raises all sorts of questions. Motoyama himself tells us that after his awakening he became aware of the karma not only of individuals, but also of larger entities such as families and nations. He discovered that he had the power to beneficially affect the karma of others. Motoymama considered this to be the most important aspect of the awakening of this chakra. Christ himself said that he could wash away the sins of the world, in other words that he could dissolve the accumulated karma of humanity.

Satyananda suggests that this chakra needs to be awakened first so that spiritual contact of a high level is established prior to releasing the karmic energies related to the other chakras. By becoming conscious at this level, it is possible to stand above karma and gain a complete understanding of it through wisdom and not the process of catharsis.

The chakras of the mind, the ajna and the sahasrara, naturally relate to the two endocrine glands within the head, the pituitary and the pineal. There is however a long-standing debate over the attribution. Some authorities attribute the ajna chakra to the pineal gland, others attribute it to the pituitary gland. This confusion is not so much a matter of disagreement as an expression of difficulty when it comes to precision at such rarefied levels of consciousness. The pineal gland is a tiny cone-shaped structure. Its real function remains a mystery. In birds the pineal gland seems to be connected with the ability to navigate using the amount of available light as a reference. Alice Bailey sets out a good case for the ajna being attributed to the pituitary gland, which is the command centre for the endocrine system as a whole. The pituitary gland is called the 'master gland' by certain yogic texts because it is said to have the power to rejuvenate the entire system. The pituitary works in conjunction with the hypothalamus to release twelve separate hormones which affect a wide range of vital functions including the repair of body tissue, patterns of sleep, breast feeding, uterine contractions during labour, and sexual maturation. In terms of physiological development the pituitary is vital. Furthermore the pituitary is divided into two distinct parts reminiscent of the two petals allocated to this chakra, the anterior and posterior lobes. My own preference after much thought is to attribute the ajna chakra to the pituitary gland and the crown chakra to the pineal gland.

The deity within this chakra is Sakti Hakini with both male and female aspects. Sakti Hakini has six heads and six arms and holds a drum, a skull, a mala, a book and makes gestures to dispel fears and grant boons. The drum symbolises the pulse of life; the skull reminds us of the need to keep the mind empty; the mala or rosary is held by the student while mantras are recited and the book symbolises wisdom. Significantly, only one deity represents the powers of this chakra as the ida, pingala and sushumna now unite to create a single current.

ORIENTATION EXERCISE

Try out your ability to visualise. The following exercise is very simple.

Sit comfortably, close your eyes and relax. Become aware of the fact that the brain is composed of two hemispheres. Visualise the number '1' in the left hemisphere and the letter 'A' in the right hemisphere. Next visualise '2' in the left hemisphere and 'B' in the right hemisphere. Continue until you reach '26' and 'Z'. Pause and enter deep relaxation. Breathe in and out through the ajna.

Now repeat the exercise by placing the letters in the left hemisphere and the numbers in the right. When you have done this you might like to compare the difference.

Now imagine the sun rising in the right hemisphere and setting in the left. Then imagine the moon rising in the left hemisphere and setting in the right. Relax and allow images that symbolise each of the hemispheres for you to spontaneously arise.

ASANAS

The ajna chakra is activated indirectly by working with the forces of the muladhara centred at the perineum. The ajna and muladhara are polar points upon the same axis. Ida, pingala and sushumna begin at muladhara and converge again at the ajna. The chakras are also linked by the same image, that of the inverted triangle which symbolises the storehouse of creative energy.

1. AWAKENING THE EYE

1. Sit with your legs crossed so that one heel presses into the area of the perineum.
2. Place your hands on your knees, keeping the spine straight.
3. Concentrate at a point between your eyebrows. Begin alternately to contract and relax your perineum upon inhalation and exhalation.
4. Next, imagine prana being absorbed into the ajna centre on the inhalation. On the exhalation imagine prana as a stream of light being radiated outwards into the universe. Chant the mantra Om, the seed mantra for this chakra.

When this exercise begins to take effect the area of your perineum will begins to feel hot; at the same time a similar sensation will be experienced between your eyebrows.

2. CLEARING THE MIND

1. Sit in a comfortable position with your hands on the floor behind you.
2. Spread your fingers so that you are aware of a slight pressure within your wrists.
3. Bring your head back and begin rythmic breathing while maintaining awareness of a point between your eyebrows. On the inhalation imagine that air in the form of white light is coming into the third eye. On the exhalation it passes out. This stimulates the pituitary gland.

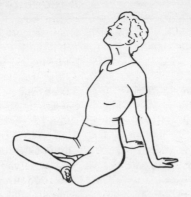

Clearing the mind

VISUALISATION: THE PLACE IN THE CLOUDS

Allow this place to dissolve and find yourself standing within an open, circular balcony. Feel a soft breeze on your face. You are standing on a balcony at the top of a high tower. You do not know how you found yourself here; it does not matter. You look out from your eyrie. Your vantage point is so high that clouds swirl beneath you. Here, you are above the clouds. The sky is bright and clear with an unfamiliar clarity. In the sky hangs a bright sun. You look down upon the clouds that hide what is below from what is above. You turn your full attention to the world far below, obscured by the clouds. Yet though your eyes cannot see, you know that far away life continues as it always has done.

Now you open the inner senses, tuning yourself to the reality of the world below. In your mind images arise, people going about their everyday lives. Below you seem to hear the cry of a new-born baby and then the last breath as someone dies to the body. Now you hear the sounds of love and now the sounds of hate. You watch in your inner mind as familiar scenes pass before you; children play, adults engage in sports, people sing, girls dance, a family sits down to a meal, a group of people raise their voices in worship.

From your vantage point you can see in every direction, you now have total vision, here in this high tower above the world. You walk to the other side of your balcony and allow the inner mind to open again. Different sounds greet you; different images fill your mind; children cry out in pain, mothers weep, young men exhalt in the sounds of war, old men wail the note of desolation.

Yet here all about you, the air is clear and bright. You are surrounded by great beauty and there is a sense of infinite peace. This place is so perfect and complete in itself. The sounds of the suffering far below trouble you. Perhaps if you were able to tell them about this place their sufferings would cease. They cannot find you, so you must find them. You make your decision.

Take one last look at the beauty and splendour of the sunlight upon the clouds. You remember every last detail so that you can tell others what you have seen. Perch upon the edge of the balcony and then, when you are ready, leap into the air.

Your descent is slow. As you fall keep reminding yourself of the need to remember what you have seen. As you fall so the light fades and dims. The sense of clarity passes. Everything seems to become hazy as you descend. There is only silence now, but you know you will find the children, the young boys, the women and the men. You hope that you have not forgotten what you came to tell them.

DREAM IMAGES

This level of consiousness transcends the dream state; it is beyond the realm of dreaming.

BACH FLOWER REMEDIES

Beech	3	Tolerance
Cerato	5	Following the inner guide
Chestnut bud	7	Being open to learning from life
Gentian	12	Acceptance
Olive	23	Trusting cosmic harmony
Walnut	33	Being able to listen to the inner voice

MUSIC

Use music to stimulate your natural ability to visualise. Enter a piece of music and allow scenes and images spontaneously to appear in the mind's eye. Try listening to *Freefall* by Malcolm Harrison, *Cascade* by Terry Oldfield or *Inner Harmony* by Arden Wilkin.

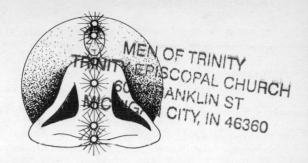

10 · THE GATEWAY OF THE VOID

THE CROWN CHAKRA: TABLE OF
CORRESPONDENCES

Location Crown of head
Sanskrit name Sahasrara, meaning 'thousandfold'
Element None applicable
Function Union
Inner state Bliss
Body parts Cerebral cortex, brain, the whole body
Gland Pineal
Malfunction Alienation
Colour Violet
Sound None applicable
Sense None applicable
Animals The risen serpent
Deities Shiva

Wise men describe it as the abode of Vishnu, and righteous men speak of it as the ineffable place of knowledge of the Atma, or the place of Liberation.

Sat-Cakra-Nirupana, verse 49

We now reach our destination. We have arrived at the final chakra and our journey is complete. We have reached the sahasrara chakra, which is represented as a multi-layered lotus of a thousand white petals. Each layer is inscribed with fifty Sanskrit letters and the petals cling closely

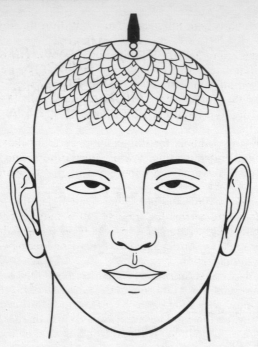

From *Kundalini Yoga for the West*

to the head to symbolise the cosmic forces which now descend like a shower upon the individual.

The sahasrara chakra is unique among the chakras. It has neither a bija mantra nor an elemental attribution. Its functions and attributes are described by its thousand petals and by the symbols contained within the pericarp of the lotus. Here we find mandalas of the sun and moon, surya and chandra respectively. The solar and lunar currents have been present throughout the journey as ida and pingala. These twin forces were absorbed into the sushumna at the brow chakra. Now their final destination is revealed. Within the mandala of the moon is a lightning-like triangle. This is described as being as fine as the hundredth part of a lotus fibre. Within this is the Nirvana-Kala. 'She is as subtle as the thousandth part of the end of a hair. She is the ever-existent Bhagavati, who is the Devata who pervades all beings. She grants divine knowledge, and is as lustrous as the light of all the suns shining at one and the same time.'[1] Within Nirvana-Kala is the para bindu which is both Shiva and Shakti. Within the bindu is the void.

These images are rather like Russian dolls residing one within the other. The difference is that of scale and meaning. We are asked to imagine the infinitesimal manifesting the infinitely great. We are confronted by the microcosmic and the macrocosmic; the void is smaller than the thousandth part of a hair yet it is also 'the chief root of Liberation'.[2]

The images and symbols for this chakra represent that which is beyond rational understanding. Words, descriptions and concepts are only pointers towards the experience of reality which defies description.

Sahasrara means thousandfold. This symbolises the totality of creation. This centre carries the total sound potential of the whole Sanskrit alphabet; fifty letters are inscribed on each of the twenty layers. The whole image is designed to convey the idea of wholeness, completion and realisation.

This centre is located four finger-breadths above the crown of the head. If you are sensitive, you can feel the presence of this chakra by holding your hand with a flat palm above the top of the head for a few moments. Even after the hand has been moved away there is a tingling or prickling sensation which emanates from above the head but can also be felt at the top of the head. This is a highly sensitive area in individuals who have opened this chakra even to a small degree. The living spiritual tradition of Tibetan Buddhism recognises this fact in the strict rules for the upbringing of its tulkus (reincarnated lamas). Lama Osel, the first recognised tulku to have been born outside Tibet, in 1985, is now being brought up with great care. One of the rules scrupulously observed by those who attend him, is that he should not be touched unnecessarily, especially at the crown of the head. This is a clear injunction to keep away from the crown chakra which would be highly sensitive and in a state of purity.[3]

It is interesting to recall that a blessing is traditionally conferred through the top of the head.

Olivia Robertson, herself highly sensitive, tells us in her book The Call of Isis that her crown chakra was triggered quite accidently. It happened in just the way that the careful Tibetan regulations were designed to avoid. She was sitting in a restaurant with a friend given to extravagant physical gestures. Her friend described the upward movement of a man reaching for fruit on a tree. She waved her arm and hand obviously too close to Olivia's head. 'As she did this I felt a light shower of power fall like a waterfall through my head. This prepared me for my later, more powerful experience.'[4]

Olivia is unusually sensitive to such things and her spontaneous response is not typical of the way in which this chakra reacts. The opening of the crown chakra usually occurs as the result of sustained spiritual development through a long period of time. This period of time is rarely confined to the space of a single lifetime. When spiritual growth is deeply ingrained with the wholeness of being, the awakening of a centre can seem to be spontaneous and practically effortless. Whereas to return to the most apt metaphor provided by Olivia's original friend, the ripened fruit falls because it is ready to do so.

The Christian tradition unconsciously recognises the same state of spiritual purity through its art and iconography. Saints and great teachers are invariably depicted with a halo of golden light about the head. This convention of religious art is now so deeply embedded that it is rarely seen for what it is: the accurate, if stylised, depiction of the awakened crown chakra itself. A halo of light is not just a piece of artistic fancy. Alice Bailey writes about the light in the head, 'The soul light penetrates into the region of the pineal gland, there it produces an irradiation of the ethers of the head. Frequently students speak of a diffused light or glow; later they may speak of seeing what appears to be like a sun.'[5]

It is not uncommon to see light fluttering around the head of someone in deep meditation. Olivia herself tells us that 'I have watched a mystic in meditation; the top of his head opened up like a volcano.'[6] When the mind is consciously involved in spiritual work the crown chakra will be active to one degree or another. When spiritual activity is integrated into daily life the crown chakra will continue gradually to open under the impetus of spiritual direction. When spiritual activity is absent the functions of the crown chakra remain dormant.

The crown chakra is called The Abode of Shiva. It is the goal of the risen Kundalini, the place where Shiva and Shakti unite. It is the place of union where the marriage is celebrated. Shakti, mother of form, rises to meet Shiva, consciousness. Two opposite yet mutually attractive powers meet and coalesce. The union of the opposites is a recurrent theme in alchemy. The partners are referred to as the king and queen or as sol and luna. These opposing forces are finally united after the completion of separate purification and transformation processes. Both alchemy and Hindu metaphysics treat the microcosm as a reflection of the macrocosm, 'As above, so below.' In other words the universal forces are particularised within the individual. The forces represented by Shiva and Shakti are both cosmic and personal at one and the same time. When these two forces are separated, human consciousness is limited by the prevailing state of duality. When Shiva and Shakti are united, human consciousness is transformed. A state of unity prevails. Ramakrishna expressed this very clearly when he wrote from personal experience. 'The distinction between the subject of consciousness and the object of consciousness is destroyed. It is a state wherein self-identity and the field of consciousness are blended in one dissoluble whole.'[7] Quite simply, the distinction between 'I' and 'you' disappears.

This state brings final liberation from the wheel of rebirth. Rebirth can serve no purpose when there is no longer any sense of self. Reincarnation is classically viewed as a means whereby consciousness is slowly released from numerous imprisoning illusions. When this task has been accomplished, consciousness is liberated or enlightened. 'That most excellent of men who has controlled his mind and known this place is never again born in the Wandering as there is nothing in the three worlds which binds him.'[8] The bindu, the point of the void, is called the chief root of liberation. The *Siva Samhita* tells us in verse 152, that 'Men as soon as they discover this most secret place become free from rebirths in this universe.'

The level of consciousness represented by the awakened crown chakra is itself the crowning achievement of the human condition. The cycle of rebirth which impels consciousness back into incarnation over and over again is finally transcended. All spiritual systems point towards an ultimate goal or final point. The goal of Yoga is union. In Hinduism, it is called moksha—liberation. In Buddhism it is called nirvana, cessation of desire. In Sufism it is called baqa, union with God. The awakening of the crown chakra is at the heart of these ultimate experiences.

The void is not itself a negation, a vacuum or absence of being. Instead it is seen to be the pure ground of being, the root of manifestation. Verse 161 of the *Siva Samhita* tells us that 'The great void, whose beginning is void, whose middle is void, whose end is void, has the brilliancy of tens of millions of suns and the coolness of tens of millions of moons. By contemplating on this, one obtains success.'

Buddhism provides us with the paradox, 'Emptiness is form, form is emptiness.' The doctrine of emptiness is the final flowering of Buddhist teaching. The realisation of emptiness is considered to be the only way to destroy the cause of suffering and to sever ignorance at the root. The direct realisation of emptiness is the means of obtaining liberation from cyclic existence. When we fully realise emptiness we clearly perceive the way in which actual phenomena exist. Our usual attitude is to believe that phenomena exist precisely as they appear to us. Then we cling to that appearance, exaggerating it quite unrealistically and all the time sowing more karmic seeds for the future.

The full realisation of the doctrine of emptiness is considered to be extremely difficult, requiring the wisdom of penetrative insight, concentration and ethical conduct. Meditation on emptiness is compared to catching a poisonous snake. It can do more harm than good if emptiness is incorrectly understood. Nihilism, the view that nothing exists, is considered to be so mistaken as to destroy all accumulated merit. Emptiness is not the realisation of non-existence but the realisation of the ultimate nature of phenomena. The realisation of emptiness is considered to be enlightenment.

It is impossible to imagine enlightenment if we ourselves are not enlightened. It is the pure and direct experience of reality. Enlightenment does not have to be an otherworldly condition. In the eastern tradition it is said that nirvana is in samsara. In the western tradition it is said that Kether is in Malkuth just as Malkuth is in Kether. This means that enlightenment is not separate from manifestation but a part of it. Enlightenment however brings an entirely different perspective to all mundane experiences.

The non-enlightened state in which most of us live is often considered to be like a prison. If we are unable to break out for ourselves, someone may break into the prison to liberate us instead. Rinpoches, Buddhist teachers, are well known for their unexpected and even bizarre behaviour that cuts right through accepted norms. There is a well-established tradition of the divine madman in Tibetan Buddhism. The Crazy Wisdom Masters, who are themselves enlightened, choose to behave in bizarre and unusual ways to break the illusions of others. There are many stories about the exploits of Drukpa Kunley and the better-known Milarepa, which serve to remind all students that enlightenment does not mean sitting crosslegged with a beatific smile. Quite the opposite in fact, for those who are enlightened have the most to give to others in the world.

It is said that the experience of physical incarnation alone provides the opportunity for enlightenment. If we do not reach an enlightened state while in the body we will not reach it in some heavenly after-life.

Exercises, techniques and methods for working with the sahasrara chakra are often withheld by teachers who are willing to give practical methods for the other chakras. Some teachers take the view that no techniques can be given because the sahasrara is beyond such a mechanical approach. It also seems likely that instructions are preserved within oral teaching traditions where there is no chance of abuse or misunderstanding. The most important factor in the awakening of the sahasrara chakra is genuine dedication, which sustains the individual through long-term spiritual practice and brings inner guidance when there is no external teacher.

Motoyama outlines the benefits and changes that awakening the sahasrara brings. When the centre begins to awaken it can bring unusually sensitive mental states. These are normally short-lived and pass. The physical body becomes healthy. The practitioner gains control over his feelings and is able to experience richer and deeper emotions with others. The powers of concentration improve, discernment becomes deeper and more reliable. The mind is freed from attachments; insight deepens. The ability to take effective action towards the fulfilment of goals increases. Psychic abilities strengthen. A direct relationship between the spiritual world and the mundane world forms at a level corresponding to the practitioner's spiritual state. The resulting freedom of mind makes it possible to exist in the realm of enlightenment while living in the world.

Motoyama personally experienced the awakening of the crown chakra. His account provides a fascinating insight into the working of the sahasrara chakra. The awakening began initially when 'a golden shining light began to enter and to leave my body through the top of my head, and I felt as if the top of my head protruded ten to twenty centimetres.' Next he saw what looked like the head of Buddha resting upon his own head. A golden white light flowed in and out through the gate at the top of the Buddha's head. 'Gradually I lost the sensation of my body, but I held a clear awareness of consciousness, of super-consciousness. I was able to hear a powerful but very tender voice resounding through the universe. Then I experienced a truly indescribable state in which my entire spiritual existence became immersed with an extraordinary calmness. After some time I felt it imperative that I return to the physical world. I descended following the same path through the gate at the top of my head.'[9]

As a result of his awakening, Motoyama discovered that he could see the outside world while in a meditative state. He could affect the bodies of others and work freely beyond karmic influences. He was also granted the blessing of union with the divine. The awakening of the sahasrara also had an effect on the other chakras. The abilities that had already been awakened within the other chakras strengthened and began to operate at higher levels. Those which had not completed their awakening developed steadily from that time on.

Motoyama's experiences led him to conclude that the awakening of the chakras is a process which must be undertaken if the soul is to evolve and find enlightenment.

The crown chakra represents the potential for enlightenment that we all possess. The sevenfold pattern represented by the chakra system is the blueprint for spiritual development.

The image of the lotus is itself a symbolic representation of the nature of the human being. The lotus roots in the mud but flowers in the air at the surface of the water. The sahasrara chakra is represented by the beautiful bloom with its many petals opening upon the head of the individual.

ORIENTATION EXERCISE

Explore what you understand by enlightenment.

ASANAS

1. HEADSTAND (SALAMBASIRSASANA)

The headstand is called the king of postures. Begin by working against a wall for support
1. Make a pad with a folded blanket.
2. Kneel facing the wall. Interlock your fingers and cup your head in the hands.
3. Place your interlocked hands firmly on the blanket. Make sure that your wrists and forearms are strong.
4. Straighten your legs and begin to walk your feet in towards the wall until your shoulders make contact with the wall. Kick up with your feet.

2. THE COMMUNION OF LIGHT

1. Sit with a straight spine.
2. Raise prana from the muladhara up to the sahasrara in a steady stream of light. Do this on a long inbreath.
3. Imagine an aperture opening at the top of your head. Let the energy stream out into the universe.
4. Visualise this energy merging with the source of all life in whatever way you conceive this.

5. On the exhalation absorb prana through the top of your head. Let it descend to the muladhara. Merge this with the pool of prana at the base of your spine by imagining the two forces coalescing into one.
6. Repeat the pattern of inhalation and exhalation.

3. THOUSAND-PETALLED LOTUS MEDITATION

1. Sit comfortably with a straight spine, rest your hands on your knees. Connect the tips of your thumbs and index fingers.
2. Imagine a lotus at the top of your head. At first its petals are tightly closed. Watch as the petals begin to unfold until the lotus is as open as possible. As the lotus opens you may hear a sound resonating internally; you may see swirling colours or feel an influx of energy through the top of the head.

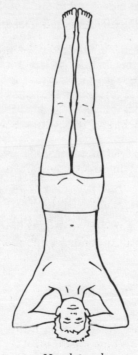

Headstand

3. Imagine that the lotus is bathed in a shaft of light. Inhale and draw energy down through the lotus. On the exhalation fill each of the chakras in descending order. If you do not feel confident enough to visualise the whole sequence, hold the energy in one chakra on the first day. Build up the sequence by adding one chakra a day at a time. It is worth spending time to master this exercise. When completed the whole body feels energised. It is helpful in awakening and cleansing the other chakras.

4. SEVEN-FOLD BREATH

1. Sit with a straight back.
2. Raise prana from the muladhara into the top of your head and exhale.
3. On next inhalation let it descend to the ajna. Hold it at the ajna by retaining your breath momentarily and exhale.
4. On the next inhalation let it fall to the vishuddi. Hold it at the vishuddi by retaining the breath momentarily and exhale.
5. Repeat with each of the chakras. When you reach the muladhara repeat the sequence and raise prana to the top of the head again. This is an excellent exercise for learning to control the flow of prana. It sharpens the inner sight and develops sensitivity to the personal flow of energies.

It is not appropriate to suggest Bach flower remedies, or music for this chakra. Instead let us end with some words from the *Siva Samhita*.

Thus constantly practising the self-luminous becomes manifest; here end all the teachings of the Guru (they can help the student no further). Henceforth he (she) must help himself (herself), they can no more increase his (her) reason or power; henceforth by the mere force of his (her) own practice he (she) must gain the Gnosis.[10]

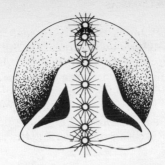

11 · THE TEMPLE OF THE LOTUS

It is important that we have the right attitude to chakra awakening. We should treat our work with reverence and care. Chakra work should not be undertaken lightly nor out of idle curiosity but out of a genuine commitment to the process of self-awareness and self-realisation.

To underline the significance and value that we place upon the process, we can make chakra awakening the focal point for ritual work. When we ritualise a process we accord it a special place in our lives. The ritual form takes the work away from the context of the mundane. It provides a space where all the senses are totally immersed in a concentrated atmosphere. We may use colour, poetry, sacred text invocation, chanting and meditation to build the Temple of the Lotus.

The preparation and necessary organisation which are required for any ritual, whether for a group or a single individual serve to focus all the energies upon the purpose of the work. If we undertake chakra work purely as an intellectual exercise we will certainly fail.

To prepare a ritual based on one of the chakras, first understand as much about the chakra as possible. Use this as the structure for your ritual. A great deal of prior organisation is required if a ritual is going to flow smoothly. Begin by deciding which chakra you wish to focus upon.

Prepare the traditional representation of the relevant chakra by painting the symbols in the appropriate colours. If you are not happy with this, select another way of representing the chakra. You might like to represent the deities of the chakra separately with a picture or other symbol. The purpose of this is to focus the whole of your energies upon the work in hand. When you have prepared these you will need to decide upon the form of the ritual and the words that will be used.

Any ritual has a number of stages: the opening, the calling of energies, the assimilation of energies, the sending forth of energies and the closing.

The following is a suggested framework for working with the muladhara chakra. It can be expanded or disregarded; it serves only as an example.

Prepare an altar with a red cloth. On the cloth there should be a candle, the prepared image for the muladhara chakra, images or symbols for the god-forms that you have chosen to work with and any other items that will be called upon.

Create a circle according to your chosen tradition. You might walk around the space three times or you might open your circle by addressing each of the quarters in turn. When your circle is created, light the candle on the altar to signify that the work has begun. Accompany this act with a statement which places your work under the auspices of the powers that you choose to work with. If you do not wish to name specific forces, open with a general statement such as, 'Let this place be opened in the name of the forces of Life and Light.'

Now you must set the work in motion by mobilising the group mind, which represents the unified mind of all those present into a single force. State your intention clearly, 'We meet to celebrate the powers of earth, to find the roots which intertwine, to establish the foundation which holds us firm.' You might like to open with appropriate music such as tribal drumming. If space permits have group dancing, which will liberate personal energies.

Bring the relevant correspondences to bear one at a time. Accompany each with poetry, prose or sacred text. Aim simply to bring out the meaning of each of the qualities of the chakra.

> Here is red, river of life,
> Attendant at birth, still at death.
> Red for our passions, red for our life,
> Roused beyond measure in our struggle to survive.

This section can be as simple or as elaborate as you wish. You could have something red on the altar as a focal point; you could light a red candle or arrange to switch the room lighting to red at this point.

Move through each of the qualities of the chakra in turn. Elemental earth can be represented by physical earth, a stone, or a small living plant. Speak about the earth which is home to us all. Draw the group mind to consider the yantra and to Airavata, the elephant of Indra.

When you have spoken on the nature of all the appropriate symbols you might like to ask a blessing from the presiding deities. Ask for whatever you feel you need from this chakra.

Now the group can move on to the more dynamic aspects of mantra and meditation. Use the bija mantra for a period of group chanting. Then move on to a guided meditation or provide a silent time for individual reflection.

Finally let each participant receive an appropriate gift. This could be a seed, a crystal or perhaps a red stone. This not only encapsulates the individual experience but also represents the energies being taken out into the world.

Close the session by reversing your opening format. Offer thanks to any supra-mundane forces that you have called into the circle and extinguish the central candle. 'Our work is done. Let us return to the outer world. Let each depart in peace one with another.'

After the ritual provide refreshment. This literally helps to bring people back to earth. It is most helpful if all the participants later prepare a written report on the work. This feedback enables individuals to explore their own reactions. The group report creates a total picture of all the shared experiences and can be helpful for planning future rituals on the other chakras. If the group meets on a regular basis the participants will naturally be able to share the longer-term effects of the work with each other.

There are no hard and fast rules for writing a ritual except that its effectiveness will be directly proportional to the effort invested in it. The preparation period can be fruitful and illuminating. It is as important as the actual experience of the ritual.

Ritual can be thought of as symbolism in activity. The circle is a dynamic three-dimensional mandala which brings symbolic values to life. It is truly the alchemical retort in which individuals may be transformed and reborn.

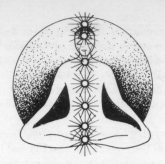

12 · THE SEVEN PALACES

I have worked with the chakras over a fifteen-year period. In that time I have explored many approaches, from the physical to the mental. I have applied traditional visualisations and created some of my own.

During one intensive period, I evolved a series of complex visualisations which centred upon a series of interconnected chambers which I entered through my inner journeys. Each chamber contained an altar set out with the appropriate symbols. Once inside the chamber I entered a deeper state of meditation and started upon another journey. This second journey often took me away from the chamber. At the end of the journey I was careful to return to the chamber before returning to waking consciousness.

I was especially interested to discover recently the Hekhalot mystical tradition. The word Hekhalot means temple or palace. The Hekhalot tradition was an early Judaic esoteric system. It made extensive use of mantra, guided visualisation, prayers, hymns, an elaborate system of correspondences and ritual practice. According to the teachings the initiate passed through a series of seven chambers. These were connected by a series of bridges and guarded by angelic forces. In order to gain admission to each succeeding chamber, the candidate had to present the appropriate seal and follow certain procedures with great care. Once inside the chamber the initiate experienced a vision, a spontaneous visualisation which revealed the secrets of the particular chamber. For instance in the seventh palace the initiate saw 'wonders and powers, majesty, and greatness, holiness, purity, terror, humility, and uprightness'.[1]

One of the central texts of the tradition describes the accomplishments and powers gained upon entry into the chambers. These include the ability to foresee the future and the ability to see the true nature of people's character. This description sounds exactly like the powers which awaken when the chakras become active. The similarities between this early Judaic system and a system of chakra awakening are quite extraordinary.

You can use the concept of the seven temples. The outline provided can be applied to each of the chakras. You will need to be experienced in visualisation and committed to your own spiritual development. You will also need a working knowledge of the relevant symbols. Don't try this exercise unless your motivation is sincere.

You stand just outside an ancient pair of doors. On the door you see inscribed the related chakra image. Until you visualise it clearly do not proceed. As you wait examine your own motives for wishing to enter the chamber.

When you are fully prepared the doors will open. You enter a huge chamber which is bathed in the glow of the appropriate colour. Seated within the chamber you will encounter the presiding deity (or deities) upon a throne(s). There may also be a table bearing relevant symbolic items. Approach the deities who will most probably examine your motives and aspirations in a deep and searching manner. This form of dialogue is often extremely cryptic. In these encounters you cannot hide or pretend; you will always be seen in a true light. The dialogue normally concludes with guidance, words of wisdom, a vision or even a symbolic gift which may help you in the outer world.

You may enter a deeper state of meditation and experience a spontaneous visualisation. If you mentally travel from the chamber, you must also return to it. Always express genuine thankfulness to the presiding deities at the end of the session. Leave the same way that you entered and close the door firmly behind you.

If you wish to work with this pattern, you must also be fully prepared to accept all responsibility for what transpires as a result.

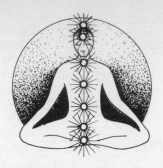

IN CONCLUSION

The purpose of this short study has been to introduce you to the chakras and to provide some basic procedures which will enable you to experience them for yourself. The discoveries you make about the chakras will also inevitably be discoveries about yourself. I wish you well on your voyage of discovery. Don't expect plain sailing all the way. Be thankful for the journey itself; it is better than the monotonous view from the safe harbour.

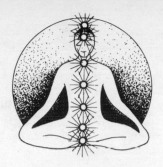

APPENDIX 1

(Reproduced with kind permission from The Theosophical Publishing House)

1. Lie flat on your back with your arms at your sides, palms upwards; enter a relaxed state. This is the shavasana (Corpse pose).

2. When relaxed and ready sit on the floor with legs extended. Place your hands palms-down on the floor beside your hips and lean slightly backwards. Flex your toes ten times; flex your ankles ten times back and forth; then draw circles in both directions with each of your feet.

3. Place your right ankle on your left thigh. Hold your ankle with your right hand, rotate your foot ten times in each direction. Repeat with your left foot on your right thigh.

4. Raise your right knee and bend it. Clasp your hands under your thigh. Straighten your leg without touching the ground. Repeat ten times with each leg.

5. Place your right foot on your left thigh. Hold your left knee with your left hand and place your right hand on top of your bent knee. Gently move the bent leg up and down. Repeat with the other leg.

6. Place the soles of your feet together and bring the heels as close to your body as possible. Allow the knees to drop as far as they are able.

7. Squat on the floor. Place your palms on your knees and walk while keeping the squatting position.

8. Sit in the original position. Extend your arms forward at shoulder height. Clench and unclench the fingers of each hand ten times. Keep

your arms extended forwards. Bend your hands back up as far as possible, then down. Repeat ten times.

9. Extend your arms forward. Drop one arm. Make a fist with your other hand. Rotate your wrists ten times in each direction.

10. Extend your arms forward palms up. Bend both your arms at the elbows and touch your shoulders with your finger tips. Repeat ten times. Then repeat with your arms extended to the sides.

11. Touch your shoulders with your fingertips. Move your elbows in circles in each direction ten times.

These exercises stimulate the joints and help to keep prana freely circulating. Source points of energy are located near the wrists and ankles. These are related to specific organs. Using these joints will keep energy flowing. The terminal points for the major meridians are located in the fingers and toes. This group of asanas is simple, yet very invigorating.

GROUP 2. ASANAS FOR REGULATING THE SUSHUMNA

These asanas work especially on the spine. They bring strength and suppleness with practice. Instructions for these postures will be found in any Yoga text book.

Concentration may be focused on a particular chakra where indicated.

1. The Mountain Pose (Tadasana).
2. Hasta Uttanasana.
3. Pada Hastasana.
4. Yoga Mudra pose (Yogasana).
5. The Pincers pose (Paschimottanasana).
6. Pada prasarita paschimottanasana.
7. The Cobra pose (Bhujangasana). Concentrate on the vishuddi chakra.
8. The Bow pose (Dhanurasana). Concentrate on the vishuddi chakra.
9. The Plough (Halasana). Concentrate on the vishuddi chakra.
10. The Fish pose (Matsyasana). Concentrate on the manipura or anahata chakra.
11. The Triangle (Trikonasana).
12. Dynamic Spinal Twist.
13. Half Spinal Twist (Arda matsyendrasana). Concentrate on the ajna chakra.
14. Spinal Twist Prostration pose (Bhu Namanasana).

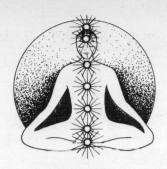

APPENDIX 2

Table of Affirmations

CHAKRA	AFFIRMATION
Muladhara	I am a part of the living universe.
	I acknowledge my connections with all living beings.
Svadisthana	I have the power to create.
	I am able to bring something new into this life.
Manipura	I am in control of my own power.
	I am able to make my own decisions.
Anahata	I feel compassion for all living beings.
Vishuddi	I express my deepest thoughts and feelings with clarity.
Ajna	I am in tune with an infinite source of guidance.
Sahasrara	I am that I am.

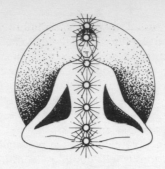

APPENDIX 3

Hiroshi Motoyama is the founder of the Institute for Religion and Parapsychology and is also a Shinto priest. He has not only experienced chakra awakening himself but has also conducted a great deal of scientific research in order to test the claims made by spiritual practitioners.

Motoyama has developed an instrument that is capable of detecting energy generated and emitted by the body. It can pick up minute electrical and magnetic changes in the immediate environment of an experimental subject. The detectors are installed inside a light-proof room which is electrostatically shielded by grounded lead sheeting embedded in the walls. The inner wall surfaces are covered in aluminium sheeting.

A round disk copper electrode and a photo-electric cell are positioned in front of the subject at the supposed level of the chakra. This location is then monitored for any change. The signals are amplified and analysed by a signal processor and a power spectrum analyser located outside the room. The subject is also monitored for respiration, ECG (measures heart rhythm) and GSR (galvanic skin response).

Motoyama has undertaken a wide range of experiments that explore the effects on people of spiritual practice. These include work on about one hundred members of the Yoga society, divided into three groups. The first group showed signs of awakened and active chakras. The second group consisted of those whose chakras were beginning to show signs of activity. The third group consisted of those whose chakras were dormant. The classification was made on the basis of Motoyama's opinion in conjunction with the subjects' own experiences.

The experiments tested disease susceptibility across the three groups and compared the functional condition of internal organs by means of electrical stimulation of viscero cutaneous reflex points.

Other experiments focused on the cardio-vascular system of yogis in comparison with individuals not in spiritual practice, and the energy emitted from the heart chakra during meditation.

Motoyama has also conducted experiments into the relationship between various PSI abilities and chakra energy.

His work forms an invaluable bridge between spiritual practice and scientific validation. It will doubtless continue to throw much-needed light onto the subtle relationship between mind, body and spirit.

Interested readers may contact the International Association for Religion and Parapsychology (I.A.R.P.):

I.A.R.P. (Main Office),
4–11–7 Inokashira,
Mitaka-shi,
Tokyo 181,
Japan.
Tel: (0422) 48–3535.

I.A.R.P. (U.S. Branch),
399 Sunset Drive,
Encinitas,
CA 92024.

Tel: (714) 753–8857.

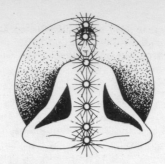

GLOSSARY

Abhayamudra The hand gesture of dispelling fear

Agni The god of fire, related to the solar plexus chakra

Airavata The elephant of Indra which emerged from the churning of the ocean, related to the base chakra

Ajna chakra The brow chakra

Akasa Spirit, ether, the fifth element

Anahata chakra The heart chakra

Anamaya kosa The food-formed sheath of the gross body

Anandakanda lotus The subsidiary centre of the heart chakra having eight petals; this is the home of the celestial wishing tree

Apana One of the five forms of prana

Applied kinesiology The science of muscle activation

Asanas The physical postures of Yoga

Astral body (or **field**) The astral aspect of the aura

Atma puri The city of the soul consisting of the physical and etheric levels together

Aura The energy field emanated by the living form

Bija mantra The seed sound of each chakra embodied in the mantra

Binah The third sephirah of the Tree of Life corresponding, jointly with Hokmah, to the ajna chakra

Bindu A point of energy ready for creation

Bodhissatva 'Wisdom-bearing'; one who is enlightened

Causal body (or **field**) The aspect of being that is based in the causal, universal level

Chakra 'Wheel'; the centres of living energy located in the subtle body

Chesed The fourth sephirah of the Tree of Life reflected along with Geburah and Tiphareth, in the heart chakra

Citrini The inner-most channel of the sushumna meridian

Dakini The Sakti or energy of the base chakra

Esoteric The inner path of spiritual practice

Etheric A level of subtle energy which interpenetrates all physical matter

Exoteric The outer path of religious observance

Gauri 'The eternal'; the great mother; deity of the throat chakra

Geburah The fifth sephirah of the Tree of Life reflected, along with Tiphareth and Chesed in the heart chakra

Goraknath A tenth-century sage and author of the *Gorakshashatakam*, a treatise on chakra awakening

Granthi Knot or junction of energy streams on the subtle body found at the base, heart and brow chakras, called the Brahma, Vishnu and Rudra knots respectively

Hakini The Sakti or energy of the brow chakra

Hod The eighth sephirah of the Tree of Life corresponding, jointly with Netzach, to the solar plexus chakra

Hokmah The second sephirah of the Tree of Life corresponding, jointly with Binah, to the ajna chakra

Ida The lunar current that starts at left side of the base chakra and terminates at the right nostril; also called Chandra or the Ganges river

Indra 'Strong and mighty'; the supreme god in the Vedic pantheon

Jalandhara banda The neck lock, used to affect the flow of Kundalini energy in the body

Kakini The Sakti or energy of the heart chakra

Karma Action, the law of cause and effect that binds consciousness to the Wheel of Rebirth

Kether The first sephirah of the Tree of Life, corresponding to the sahasrara chakra

Kirlian photography A photographic technique that reveals the energy emanated by living forms

Kundalini The serpent power dormant within the base chakra

Lakini The Sakti or energy of the manipura chakra

Lalana chakra A secondary chakra in the subtle body, in the region of the brain stem

Makara A crocodile-like creature related to the svadisthana chakra

Malkuth The tenth sephirah of the Tree of Life corresponding to the base chakra

Manipura chakra The solar plexus chakra

Meditation The discipline of controlling the mind in order to bring about a state of liberation

Mental body (or **field**) **The mental aspect of the aura**

Meridian A channel that conducts pranic energies; also called a nadi

Meru The spine in the microcosm, Mount Meru as centre of the universe in the macrocosm

Moksha The state of liberation according to the Hindu tradition

Mulabanda The root lock, applied to affect the flow of Kundalini energy in the body

Muladhara chakra The base chakra

Nadi (Nadir) A channel that conducts pranic energies; also called a meridian

Netzach The seventh sephirah of the Tree of Life corresponding, jointly with Hod, to the solar plexus chakra

Nirvana The state of liberation according to the Buddhist tradition

Niyama Virtuous conduct consisting of five practices

Otz Chim The Tree of Life; the central glyph of the Qabalah

Padma The lotus, a symbolic description of a chakra

Padmasana The lotus position, the classic pose for meditation
Pingala The solar current originating at the right side of the base chakra, terminating at the left nostril; also called Surya or the Yamuna River
Prana The universal life force that permeates all living things
Pranamaya kosa The vital or etheric sheath
Pranayama The practice of controlling the flow of breath
Privithi The elemental symbol of earth, also a goddess
Qabalah The esoteric aspect of Judaism
Rakini The Sakti or energy of the sacral chakra
Sahasrara chakra The crown chakra
Sakti (Shakti) The feminine aspect of the divine in manifestation
Samana One of the five forms of prana
Sat-Cakra-Nirupana The major Sanskrit text dealing with the chakras
Sephirah (plural **Sephiroth**) The ten Holy Emanations of the Qabalistic Tree of Life
Shiva The masculine aspect of the divine in manifestation
Sushumna The spinal meridian identified with the governor vessel
Svadisthana chakra The sacral chakra
Tantra An esoteric path leading to enlightenment
Tiphareth The sixth sephirah of the Tree of Life corresponding, along with Geburah and Chesed, to the heart chakra
Udana One of the five forms of prana
Uddiyana banda The diaphragm lock applied to affect the flow of Kundalini energies in the body
Upanishad Hindu scriptures
Uyana One of the five forms of prana
Vajra The secondmost channel of the sushumna meridian; also the name applied to a ritual sceptre in the form of a thunderbolt
Vara (Varada) A hand gesture that symbolises the granting of boons
Vayu God of the winds
Vedas Earliest Hindu scriptures
Vishnu The divine preserver
Vishuddi chakra The throat chakra
Yama Abstention from non-virtuous conduct
Yesod The ninth sephirah of the Tree of Life corresponding to the sacral chakra

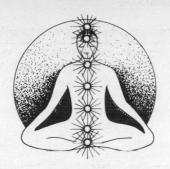

NOTES AND REFERENCES

CHAPTER 1. THE LANDSCAPE OF SUBTLE ENERGIES

1. Alice Bailey, *A Compilation on Sex*, p. 28.
2. See *The Body Electric* by Thelma Moss for an autobiographical account of developments in the field of Kirlian photography.
3. Gopi Krishna, *Kundalini, The Evolutionary Energy in Man*, pp. 38 and 241.
4. Alice Bailey, *The Light of the Soul*, p. 172.

CHAPTER 2. APPROACHING THE GATES

1. Alice Bailey, *The Soul The Quality of Life*, p. 172.
2. Alice Bailey, *A Treatise on White Magic*, p. 202.
3. B. K. S. Iyengar, *Light on Pranayama*.
4. Crystal elixirs are available from Crystal World, Anubis House, Creswell Drive, Ravenstone, Leics. E6 2AG, England.

CHAPTER 5. THE GATEWAY OF THE MOON

1. P. Shuttle & P. Redgrove, *The Wise Wound*, p. 137.
2. Alice Bailey, *A Compilation on Sex*, p. 67.

CHAPTER 6. THE GATEWAY OF THE SUN

1. Leslie Kenton, *The Bioenergetic Diet*.
2. Alexandra David-Neel, *Magic and Mystery in Tibet*, p. 163.
3. Alexandra David-Neel, *Magic and Mystery in Tibet*, p. 161.

CHAPTER 7. THE GATEWAY OF THE WINDS

1. Gorree & Barbier, *The Love of Christ*.
2. Prabhavananda, *The Spiritual Heritage of India*, p. 150.
3. Gopi Krishna, *Kundalini, The Evolutionary Energy in Man*, p. 207.
4. Gopi Krishna, *Kundalini, The Evolutionary Energy in Man*, p. 209.
5. *The Upanishads*, trans. Max Muller, Katha Upanishad 11 6.15.
6. Hiroshi Motoyama, *Theories of the Chakras*, p. 249.

CHAPTER 8. THE GATEWAY OF TIME AND SPACE

1. Tolkien, *The Silmarillion* p. 17.
2. John Diamond, *Speech and Language and the Power of the Breath*. According to John Diamond, there is a relationship between the following sounds and the meridians.
3. Hiroshi Motoyama, *Theories of the Chakras*, p. 251.

SOUND	MERIDIAN	SOUND	MERIDIAN
P, B	Stomach	T, D, N	Governing vessel
M	Large intestine	L	Central
F, V	Small intestine	Y	Gall bladder
R	Triple warmer	K, G	Kidney
S, Z	Heart	H	Spleen
SH, CH, J	Circulation and sex	Q	Lung
TH	Liver		

4. Hiroshi Motoyama, *Theories of the Chakras*, p. 250.
5. Hiroshi Motoyama, *Theories of the Chakras*, p. 251.
6. *Journal of the International Association for Religion and Parapsychology*, Vol 3, No. 1, 'Western and Eastern Medical Studies of Pranayama and Heart Control.'

CHAPTER 10. THE GATEWAY OF THE VOID

1. Trans. Sir John Woodroffe, *Sat-Cakra-Nirupana*, verse 47.
2. Trans. Sir John Woodroffe, *Sat-Cakra-Nirupana*, verse 42.
3. Vicki Mackenzie, *Reincarnation, the Boy Lama*, p. 159.
4. Olivia Robertson, *The Call of Isis*, p. 55.
5. Alice Bailey, *A Treatise on White Magic*, p. 106.
6. Olivia Robertson, *The Call of Isis*.
7. Sri Ramakrishna, *The Great Master Saradananda*, p. 364.
8. Arthur Avalon, *The Serpent Power*, verse 45.
9. Hiroshi Motoyama, *Theories of the Chakras*, p. 254.
10. *Siva Samhita*

CHAPTER 12. THE SEVEN PALACES

1. Dr. Deidre Green, *The Hermetic Journal*, No. 31, The Seven Palaces in Early Jewish Mysticism.

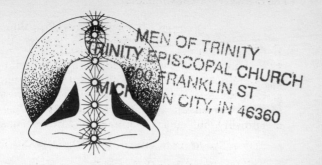

BIBLIOGRAPHY

Achterberg, Jean, *Imagery in Healing*, Shambala, 1985.

Allen, Marcus, *Tantra for the West*, Whatever Publishing (San Raphael, California), 1981.

Avalon, Arthur, *The Serpent Power*, Dover Publications, 1974.

Bailey, Alice, *The Soul, The Quality of Life*, Lucis Publishing Company, 1974.

Bailey, Alice, *A Treatise on White Magic*, Lucis Publishing Company, 1974.

Bailey, Alice, *A Compilation on Sex*, Lucis Publishing Company, 1980.

Bentov, Itzhak, *Stalking the Wild Pendulum*, Fontana, 1979.

Conze, E, *Buddhist Scriptures*, Penguin, 1984.

Dass, Ram, *The Only Dance There Is*, Anchor Books, 1974.

David-Neel, Alexandra, *Initiations and Initiates in Tibet*, Rider, 1970.

Davis, Mikol & Lane, Earl, *Rainbows of Life*, Harper Colophon Books, 1978.

Dowman, Keith, *The Divine Madman, The Sublime Life and Songs of Drukpa Kunley*, Dawn Horse Press (California), 1980.

Durckheim, Karlfried, Graf, *Hara, the Vital Centre of Man*, Unwin Hyman, 1988.

Evans-Wentz, W. Y. *Tibetan Yoga and Secret Doctrines*, Oxford University Press, 1973.

Fortune, Dion, *The Mystical Qabalah*, Ernest Benn Ltd. 1976.

Gach, Michael & Marco, Carolyn, *Acu-Yoga*, Japan Publications Inc. 1981.

Guenther, H. & Trungpa, C. *The Dawn of Tantra*, Shambala Dragon, 1975.

Happold, F. C. *Mysticism*, Pelican, 1963.

Humphrey, Naomi, *Meditation the Inner Way*, Aquarian, 1987.

Iyengar, B. K. S. *Light on Yoga*, Schocken Books, 1977.

Iyengar, B. K. S. *Light on Pranayama*, Unwin, 1981.

Judith, Anodea, *Wheels of Life*, Llewellyn Publications, 1987.

Kenton, Leslie, *Bioenergetic Diet*, Arrow Books, 1986.

Keyes, Laurel Elizabeth, *Toning, the Creative Power of the Voice*, DeVorss & Company, 1978.

Kilner, W. *The Human Aura*, University Books, 1965.

Klimo, Jon, *Channelling*, Aquarian Press, 1988.

Krishna, Gopi. *Kundalini, the Evolutionary Energy in Man*, Shambala Publications Inc, 1970.

Leadbeater, C. W. *The Chakras*, Theosophical Publishing House, 1980.
Lethbridge, T. C. *E.S.P. Beyond Time and Distance*, Sidgwick and Jackson, 1974.
Lowen, Alexander, *Bioenergetics*, Penguin Books, 1975.
Lu K'uan Yu, *Taoist Yoga*, Rider and Co. 1970.
Mackenzie, Vicki, *Reincarnation, the Boy Lama*, Bloomsbury, 1989.
McLean, Adam, *The Hermetic Journal*, No. 31.
Mead, G. R. S. *The Doctrine of the Subtle Body in Western Tradition*, Stuart and Watkins, 1967.
Mookerjee, Ajit, *Kundalini*, Thames and Hudson, 1982.
Mookerjee, Ajit, *The Tantric Way*, New York Graphic Society, 1977.
Moore, Rickie, *A Goddess in my Shoes*, Humanics New Age, 1988.
Moss, Thelma, *The Body Electric*, Granada, 1981.
Motoyama, Hiroshi, *Theories of the Chakras: Bridge to Higher Consciousness*, Theosophical Publishing House, 1988.
Parfitt, Will, *The Living Qabalah*, Element Books, 1988.
Powell, A. E. *The Etheric Double*, Theosophical Publishing House, 1979.
Radha Sivananda Swami, *Kundalini Yoga for the West*, Shambala Publications Inc. 1978.
Radice, Betty, ed., *The Upanishads*, Penguin, 1985.
Rawson, Philip, *Tantra*, Thames and Hudson, 1973.
Rendel, Peter, *Introduction to the Chakras*, 1977.
Robertson, Olivia, *The Call of Isis*, Cesara Publications, 1975.
Ross & Wilson, *Anatomy and Physiology in Health and Illness*, Churchill Livingstone, 1987.
Satprem, *Sri Aurobindo, or the Adventure of Consciousness*, Harper and Row, 1968.
Satyananda, Paramahamsa, *Pranya Vidya*, International Yoga Fellowship, 1976.
Scott, Mary, *Kundalini in the Physical World*, Routledge & Kegan Paul, 1983.
Sherwood, Keith, *Chakra Therapy for Personal Growth and Healing*, Llewellyn Publications, 1988.
Shuttle, P. & Redgrove, P. *The Wise Wound*, Paladin, 1978.
Silburn, Lilian, *Kundalini, Energy of the Depths*, State University of New York Press, 1988.
Siva Samhita, The Oriental Book Reprint Cooperation, 1975.
Sri Ramakrishna, *The Great Master Saradananda*, Madras.
Stutley, Margaret & James, eds., *Harper's Dictionary of Hinduism*, Harper and Row, 1977.
Tansley, David, *Radionics, Interface with the Ether-Fields*, Health Science Press, 1979.
Tansley, David, *Radionics and the Subtle Anatomy of Man*, Health Science Press, 1976.
Thie, John F. *Touch for Health*, DeVorss & Co. 1979.
Tolkien, J. R. R. *The Silmarillion*, Unwin Hyman, 1977.
Vollmar, Klausbernd, *Journey Through the Chakras*, Gateway Books, 1987.
Watson, Andrew & Drury, Neville, *Healing Music*, Nature and Health Books, 1987.
Wilhelm, Richard, *The Secret of the Golden Flower*, Arkana, 1974.
Wood, Ernest, *Yoga*, Pelican Books, 1969.

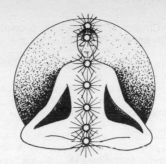

INDEX